The Science
of
Staying Young

JOHN E. MORLEY, M.D.
AND
SHERI R. COLBERG, PH.D.

New York Chicago San Francisco Lisbon London Madrid Mexico City
Milan New Delhi San Juan Seoul Singapore Sydney Toronto

Library of Congress Cataloging-in-Publication Data

Morley, John E.
    The science of staying young / John E. Morley and Sheri R. Colberg.
       p.   cm.
    Includes bibliographical references.
    ISBN 13: 978-0-07-149283-6 (alk. paper)
    ISBN 10: 0-07-149283-6 (alk. paper)
    1. Longevity.   I. Colberg, Sheri, 1963–   II. Title.

RA776.75 M67   2007
613.2—dc22   2007030606

For my older friends and patients, who have been my best teachers, and my

grandchildren (Amanda, Conor, Katelyn, Nicole, and Paige), who are my

inspiration and keep me aging successfully

—*John Morley*

For Ray Ochs, my best friend, husband, and partner in

feeling and looking younger than we are

—*Sheri Colberg*

1 2 3 4 5 6 7 8 9 10 11 12 13 14 15 16 17 18 19 20 21   FGR/FGR   0 9 8 7

ISBN 978-0-07-149283-6
MHID   0-07-149283-6

Interior design by Think Design Group

McGraw-Hill books are available at special quantity discounts to use as premiums and sales promotions, or for use in corporate training programs. For more information, please write to the Director of Special Sales, Professional Publishing, McGraw-Hill, Two Penn Plaza, New York, NY 10121-2298. Or contact your local bookstore.

Contents

Preface

Your Lifelong Journey

"To know how to grow old is the master work of wisdom, and one of the most difficult chapters in the great art of living."
—*Henri-Frédéric Amiel (1821–1881)*

The poet lyrically invites us to, "Grow old along with me; the best is yet to be." In return, the cynic responds, "What damn fool said that?" Regardless of whether you are more of a poet or a cynic, it is doubtlessly clear to all of you reading this book that aging is *not* for sissies. The process of getting older, although inevitable, can be a difficult one both physically and mentally. But take heart, because you can do many things to keep yourself feeling and looking younger than you really are.

Our purpose in writing this book is to share with you ten simple, but critical, steps for maintaining an optimal quality of life throughout your lifetime, regardless of your current age and the genes that you inherited. In fact, if you start to follow the suggestions in this book, within days and weeks you will likely experience the following, no matter how old you are:

- An upsurge in your energy levels
- An enhanced enjoyment of your life and daily activities
- A noticeable increase in the sharpness of your mind
- A stronger sex drive

While these results will be more immediate, other benefits, like a fine wine, will take more time to fully appreciate—months, years, or even a lifetime.

This book is your passport to aging successfully and feeling your best at any age. Like anyone with a passport, however, you get to choose where you go with it. Throughout, we point out the minimum that needs to be done at any particular stop along the way, as well as what we consider to be optimal. Wherever possible, we also give you alternate choices since there is no single way to age gracefully. The path you choose to optimize your physical and mental journey through the rest of your life should be the one that works best for you.

What This Book Is *Not* About

At the outset, it is important to stress what this book is *not* about. First, we're not here to promise you the impossible or to convince you to make sweeping and dramatic changes in your current lifestyle. Alternately, our goal is to help you recognize where even small improvements can have the greatest impact on your overall health. For example, one of us (Dr. John) is inherently a physical sloth with an epicurean delight in gourmet food and wine, while the other (Dr. Sheri) is a more traditional believer in the physical and mental benefits of a healthy diet and regular physical activity. For her, exercise results more reliably in an endorphin high, while he questions whether exercise is anything more than "the ultimate experience in masochism." Regardless of whose viewpoint you more closely identify with, accepting the idea that participation in at least some exercise is essential will benefit you immensely.

The second thing that this book is *not* about is life extension—that is, increasing your longevity. We both fervently believe that enjoyment of life (by adding quality to your life) is far more important than simply racking up additional years. Living longer when plagued by debilitating illnesses, immobility, or a loss of independence is not necessarily a gift. Over a quarter of a century ago, Professor James Fries at Stanford University first suggested that each individual's goal should not be an extension of life, but rather a higher quality of life. Living well and feeling good enough to do whatever you want to do throughout your lifetime is priceless. If you follow our suggestions in this book, you will likely come closer to this optimal goal, and you may even end up with a better *and* a longer life.

Understanding How Your Body Changes over Time

The changes that your body undergoes over time are complex and involve both normal physiological and disease processes. In general, your body experiences very gradual and subtle alterations in how well its different systems—such as breathing, digestion, and sexual ability—function over time. Human cells apparently have a limited number of times that they can split and reproduce. Once your cells slow their rate of turnover, these subtle changes start to accelerate. Unfortunately, such effects are often inseparable from the onset of chronic diseases like heart disease and cancer.

Whether a true dichotomy exists between health problems caused by natural aging or by disease, however, is largely irrelevant. If we could find a way to prevent all diseases from occurring, our lives would eventually end at some point when our cells reached their maximal life span. But attempting to achieve greater longevity by preventing and effectively treating diseases that can shorten your life is entirely relevant and a central purpose of this book. For example, the density of bones peaks somewhere around twenty-five years of age, after which time they may start to lose some stored calcium and other minerals. Muscles fibers, too, must be routinely used to prevent excess losses of muscle with each passing decade. However, this is an area where regular physical activity will likely be beneficial and have an immediate effect. Likewise, a lesser ability to absorb adequate amounts of vitamins and minerals from foods may be almost entirely countered by dietary improvements that are easy to implement (as outlined in later steps in this book).

No Easy Fixes

The first bestselling book on aging was written in the thirteenth century by Roger Bacon. It gave the following rules for success: controlled diet, proper rest, exercise, moderation in lifestyle, good hygiene, and inhalation of the breath of a virgin. We can attest to all of these recommendations—with the exception of the last one. However, virtually every bestselling book about aging written since that time has included one or more modern equivalents of the "breath of a virgin."

By way of example, Dr. Deepak Chopra, one of America's spiritual gurus with an interest in holistic healing, wrote a seemingly sensible book not long ago that included a mention of an Ayurvedic herb purported to extend life. Initially, Dr. John had been recommending Chopra's book to his older patients. But he stopped doing so when they started complaining that he was holding out on them and asked if he would please tell them where to get these precious herbs. When asked if they were walking up ten flights of stairs a day or changing their diets for the better, as Dr. John routinely recommends, they invariably replied, "No, doctor, that's too hard. I just want the herb."

What This Book Has to Offer

Our book has no virginal breath to offer you. We are alternately offering something even better: an innovative program with easily implemented steps that actually work to help you feel, look, and act younger for longer. You may not be preventing, reversing, or even slowing your aging per se, but following the steps outlined in this book will invariably make your journey through the rest of your life from this point forward as enjoyable—and as disease free—as humanly possible.

Our proactive approach to your successful aging contains ten easy-to-follow steps aimed at understanding, preventing, controlling, and reversing most health problems that can make you feel older or shorten your life. Our program explains the best foods to eat, why alcohol can be beneficial (and how much to drink), what types of exercise are important, which hormones are most likely to enhance your vigor, how to keep your mind sharp, and why weight loss may not be advisable at certain ages. It additionally gives you the knowledge to keep your heart healthy, prevent cancer, thicken up your bones, keep your joints limber, and stay on your feet.

Remarkably, your own fate has never been more in your own hands. We sincerely hope that you will choose to use this passport to immediate better health and a successful rest-of-your-life.

Acknowledgments

First, we would like to acknowledge that this book is based on many articles that originally appeared in *Aging Successfully* and that were written by Dr. John Morley. This newsletter is edited by Nina Tumosa, Ph.D.

Next, we would like to thank our families for putting up with both of us during the book-writing process. In particular, Dr. John thanks his wife, Pat, who put up with his long working hours, and the faculty, staff, and residents of the Division of Geriatrics at Saint Louis University and the Veterans Administration. Dr. Sheri also gives her thanks, apologies, and love to her husband, Ray, and her three sons, Alex, Anton, and RayJ, who did not get to see quite enough of her until this book was finished.

We would also like to thank all the hardworking individuals at McGraw-Hill who, with their feedback and dedication, have made this book into a program that everyone easily can follow to live long and well, particularly our editor, Johanna Bowman. Our appreciation also goes out to the individuals who read through this book and gave us feedback, including Etta Vinik, M.A., Lisa Little, and Joe Jansen.

Next, we would like to acknowledge Patrick Ochs of Och Tree Productions who created the exercise illustrations found in this book and thank him for coming through for Dr. Sheri yet again. His skillfully crafted creations are much appreciated.

Finally, where would we even be without our persistent and very capable literary agent, Linda Konner? Thanks again for believing in our concept and giving us encouragement every step along the way.

Introduction

Start on the Steps to Successful Aging

> "To resist the frigidity of old age, one must combine the body, the mind, and the heart. And to keep these in parallel vigor one must exercise, study, and love."
>
> —*Charles-Victor de Bonstettin (1867–1947)*

How many times have you heard people blame all of their aches and pains on "getting old"? Both of us have heard it frequently even from people in their thirties and forties. Maybe you have also used it as an explanation for why you feel achy when you stand up after sitting too long or for why you're now experiencing a "middle-age spread" when you've never had problems keeping your weight down before. Many of these types of symptoms so commonly attributed to getting older may actually be reversible or preventable, meaning that they're likely not inevitable consequences of aging at all.

Using Our Ten-Step Program

Once you have read through all of the steps and begun implementing some of our suggestions into your daily life, you're certain to start experiencing some noticeable health benefits, many of which will be readily apparent in six months or less. Whether you follow all of the steps depends on your own unique situation and your individual preferences. If nothing else, at least you will have gained the knowledge base to make informed decisions about what to do to optimize both your current health and how well you look and feel from here on out.

To make it easier to tell the difference between honest-to-goodness effects of getting older (which you can only minimally affect) and health problems resulting from other causes (which you may be able to do something about), we're going to tell you some of the more important questions to ask about aging successfully and where to find the answers in the ten steps of this book:

• Why don't French women get fat? (Step 1)
• How much fish should you eat, and when do you need fish oil? (Step 1)
• How much alcohol is good, and does it have to be red wine? (Step 1)
• Can a super-antioxidant supplement slow down aging? (Step 1)
• Is walking the only exercise you need to do? (Step 2)
• Why is it important to practice balancing on one leg? (Step 2)
• Can exercise really keep you from getting gray hair? (Step 2)
• Why is vitamin D likely the most important antiaging hormone? (Step 3)
• Is testosterone good for both men and women? (Step 3)
• Is estrogen really back in vogue again? (Step 3)
• Is it possible to reverse Alzheimer's disease? (Step 4)
• Do crossword puzzles and Sudoku really keep your mind sharp? (Step 4)
• Why does attending church help you live longer, when listening to a televangelist doesn't? (Step 4)
• Why is weight loss bad for you as you age? (Step 5)
• Can you still look muscular once you reach fifty? (Step 5)
• How does eating dark chocolate help prevent heart attacks? (Step 6)
• When is "bad" cholesterol really good for your heart? (Step 6)
• Is it possible to lower your chances for breast or prostate cancer? (Step 7)

- Can preventing diabetes affect your risk for colon cancer? (Step 7)
- Does regular exercise prevent or reverse thinning bones? (Step 8)
- Can chondroitin and glucosamine make your arthritic joints feel like new? (Step 8)
- Can hip fractures resulting from falls be prevented? (Step 9)
- Why will spontaneous physical activity (SPA) help you live longer and better? (Step 9)
- Can taking too many medications cause more problems than it solves? (Step 10)
- When should you see a doctor who specializes in aging? (Step 10)

Our proactive approach to staying and feeling young longer is largely focused on preventing, controlling, and reversing many chronic conditions that can cause you to lose your vitality or your good health. These goals can largely be accomplished through a healthier lifestyle and earlier medical intervention. The ten simple steps, along with action steps given throughout the book, will help you easily implement changes into your life. The ones that we consider to be most important for you to immediately implement into your life are listed as "Action Steps for Better Health" in each chapter. As you read through this book, you can start implementing the suggestions given in each step as you go—without necessarily waiting until you reach the end of the book. For example, as soon as you learn how healthy fish is for both your heart and your brain, you can start eating more of it, while avoiding the types of fish with too much mercury in them.

Action Steps for Better Health Tip #1

For immediately improving your health, start implementing the suggestions given in each step as you go, without waiting until you reach the end of this book.

Being Healthy at Any Age

Promoting good health is best when done over a lifetime, but you can still start implementing healthful practices at any time to increase your odds of longer survival and a stronger, healthier body. You can always gain some of the health promotion benefits, regardless of your current age, but the sooner you get started, the better your results will likely be.

It is important to note, however, that some guidelines change as time passes, and what is appropriate for you at twenty years of age may not be when you reach forty, sixty, or older. For general guidelines to optimal health at any age, consult the sidebar that follows, which was developed by Dr. John for the *Aging Successfully* magazine produced by Saint Louis University and the Saint Louis Veterans Administration.

A Guide to Optimal Health over Your Lifetime

0–40 Years

1. Exercise regularly.
2. Avoid obesity.
3. Ingest adequate calcium.
4. Eat nutritious foods, including fish.
5. Wear your seat belt.
6. Drink in moderation after age 21, and do not smoke.
7. Get your vaccinations.
8. Drive at a safe speed (once you get your driver's license).
9. Avoid violence and illicit drugs.
10. Do a monthly breast self-exam (females, after menstruation begins).

40–60 Years

1. Exercise regularly.
2. Avoid obesity.
3. Ingest adequate calcium and vitamin D.

4. Eat fish.
5. Wear your seat belt.
6. Drink in moderation, and do not smoke.
7. Have your blood pressure checked.
8. Get your cholesterol and glucose checked.
9. Screen for breast and colon cancer, high blood pressure, and diabetes.
10. Get regular Pap smears (females).
11. Have regular mental activity and socialize.
12. Avoid taking too many medicines.
13. Consider hormone replacement (males and females).

60–80 Years
1. Exercise regularly, including balance and resistance exercises.
2. Avoid weight loss.
3. Ingest adequate calcium and vitamin D.
4. Eat fish.
5. Wear your seat belt.
6. Drink in moderation, and do not smoke.
7. Screen for breast and colon cancer, high blood pressure, osteoporosis, and diabetes.
8. Get your cholesterol checked.
9. Have flu, pneumococcal, and possibly herpes zoster vaccinations.
10. Get regular Pap smears (females).
11. Have regular mental activity and socialize.
12. Avoid taking too many medicines.

80+ Years
1. Exercise regularly, including balance and resistance exercises.
2. Avoid weight loss.
3. Ingest adequate calcium and vitamin D.
4. Be screened for osteoporosis.

(continued)

5. Wear your seat belt.
6. Drink in moderation, and do not smoke.
7. Have your blood pressure checked.
8. Do monthly breast self-exams (females).
9. Have flu and pneumococcal vaccinations.
10. Make your home safety proof to prevent falls; if you are unsteady, use a cane and consider hip protectors.
11. Have regular mental activity, socialize, and avoid being depressed.
12. Avoid taking too many medicines.
13. Keep doing what you are doing right.

Can You Alter Your Life Expectancy?

There is no doubt that life expectancies have risen dramatically in many areas of the world during the past century. The average life span of anyone in an industrialized nation has increased by over thirty years due to improvements in public health, vaccinations, and disease prevention since the turn of the last century. Fewer people have been negatively impacted by uncontained outbreaks of infectious diseases such as smallpox that can be vaccinated against or from easily treatable conditions like pneumonia.

Rising longevity along with falling fertility rates are the primary reasons for the recent aging of the world's population in more affluent areas such as the United States and Europe, recently causing their citizens to start "graying" rapidly. Only countries like France that have tax credits for child care and other government-based programs to support the expansion of younger populations are starting to balance out the young and older populations more effectively.

Will Life Expectancies Continue to Increase?

It's highly unlikely that life expectancies will continue to rise equivalently in the coming decades. The approximate ten million cells in your body have a limited life span, meaning they can only divide a certain number of times (their method of reproducing) before they begin to age and stop reproducing, a phenomenon known as the Hayflick limit after its discoverer, Dr. Leonard Hayflick. The human life-span limit is believed to be close to 125 years, although very few of us reach that ripe old age.

Why don't more of us make it to even a hundred years? The reasons are varied, but nearly all of us experience life-shortening disease states while our cells still have the capacity to keep dividing and re-creating themselves, ones such as heart disease and cancer. Thus, while it may not be possible to change your cells' pre-programming, prevention or better treatment of these diseases, if they occur, will allow you to come closer to your unique Hayflick limit.

In the United States, the average person lives into his or her seventies, at least four decades short of the potential maximum age. Once you reach the age of seventy, your life expectancy is greater than average (see Table I.1), particularly if you are healthy. If you live to be eighty, you can revel in the fact that you have outlived most of your physicians.

TABLE I.1 Life Expectancy for Anyone Reaching the Age of 70

Average Years Left to Live

Men						
Age	70	75	80	85	90	95
Healthy	18.0	14.2	10.8	7.9	5.8	4.3
Average	12.4	9.3	6.7	4.7	3.2	2.3
Frail	6.7	4.9	3.3	2.2	1.5	1.0
Women						
Age	70	75	80	85	90	95
Healthy	21.3	17.0	13.0	9.6	6.8	4.8
Average	15.7	11.9	8.6	5.9	3.9	2.7
Frail	9.5	6.8	4.6	2.9	1.8	1.7

How Old Are You Really?

"My birth certificate was in the Bible and the goat ate the Bible."
—Leroy Robert "Satchel" Paige (1906–1982)

Your chronological age is your actual age in years from the date of your birth; however, what really matters is your physiological, or biological, age. This latter age is an estimate of your well-being and general health compared to others of your age and to those who are younger or older than you. People who are limited by health problems at fifty are considered to be biologically older, while robust eighty-year-olds are "super-agers."

While it would be great if you could easily calculate your likely life span, doing so is actually a complex process that we just briefly touch on in this step. To determine your biological age, you need to take into account how long your close relatives have lived (e.g., parents, grandparents, and siblings), your health at birth, your rate of tissue aging, your attitudes and coping skills, and your current and past lifestyles.

Action Steps for Better Health Tip #2

You're only as old as you feel. Your biological age is a much greater determinant of your longevity and vitality than your chronological age, so take control of your health sooner rather than later to lower the age that really matters and to feel younger.

How Much Your Genes Matter

Your genes apparently determine 20 to 50 percent of how long you will be alive. In the United States, women live about five years longer than men. For women, the most accurate predictor of their genetic effect is chronological age at menopause. The mean age of menopause for American women is fifty-two years, but in general, the later that menopause occurs, the longer a woman will live. If you have not reached that time of your life yet, your mother's age at menopause will give you a reasonable estimate of your expected menopause and probable genetic age.

In actuality, your genetic age is neither a direct determination by your mother and father, nor the direct result of the gene mixture they gave you. Rather, your endowment with specific antiaging genes may enhance your longevity. For instance, if you have the certain genes associated with a more normal blood pressure, you have a better chance of living longer. Similarly, if you inherited certain genes associated with better fat metabolism, you will age more slowly that someone with other genetic characteristics that cause the body to deal with fat less effectively, which may be associated with increased heart attacks and a greater risk of Alzheimer's disease.

Other genes that have been suggested as players in aging include those associated with how well you deal with stress, or your body's hormonal response to stress; your levels of growth hormone; how well your body controls levels of inflammation, which are known to contribute to heart disease and diabetes; and your cells' ability to produce energy. Mutations in DNA found in your cells' powerhouses, the mitochondria, may be associated with faster aging and the onset of diseases such as diabetes. While new longevity genes, or gerontogenes, are being discovered at an amazingly rapid rate, until the time that gene therapies are available to alter your genes for the better, it may not be that important, or comforting, to know what types of genes you inherited.

Action Steps for Better Health Tip #3

Your genes apparently determine 20 to 50 percent of how long you are going to live, which really means that 50 to 80 percent of your aging may be more directly under your control. Learn how to positively alter your internal and external influences, such as stress management, to enhance your longevity.

Biomarkers of Tissue and Organ Aging

Different tissues and organs change over time at varying rates, so enhancing their function by taking the steps in this book will likely slow your rate of biological aging and, in some cases, even reverse it. Some of the more common biomarkers for aging that you can have tested are listed in the following sidebar. Unfortunately, most of them you can't do on your own, but by learning more about them, you will at least know which tests to consider having at some point.

Biomarkers Indicative of Biological Aging

- Cardiovascular function (blood pressure, heart strength)
- Metabolic activity (blood glucose and cholesterol levels)
- Maximal aerobic capacity (exercise stress testing)
- Muscular strength (hand grip strength)
- Breathing capacity (forced vital capacity and expiratory volume)
- Bone mineral density
- Skin elasticity
- Mental function (cognitive abilities, including memory)
- Systemic inflammation (measured by markers in blood)
- Reaction time (nerve conduction velocity)

Control Your Blood Pressure. An easily measured biomarker of aging is your systolic blood pressure, which is the first number in a blood pressure reading, such as 130 in a reading of 130/85. A normal blood pressure never has a systolic value of more than 120, but elevations in systolic pressure are more common the older you get (more on the effects of high blood pressure and how to control it in Step 6). Systolic pressures reflect the elasticity of your arteries, or how well they expand when your heart pumps blood into them. The longer your value stays in a normal or near normal range, the younger your vessels are acting. Either have your pressure measured at your next doctor's visit, or step into the nearest pharmacy and measure it yourself for free. Although drugstore testing is less accurate, it still gives you a ballpark idea of your systolic reading.

Action Steps for Better Health Tip #4

Certain biomarkers of biological aging can let you know whether you're doing better or worse than your chronological age would indicate. Consider having your blood pressure, blood glucose and cholesterol levels, maximal aerobic capacity, breathing capacity, bone mineral density, or any combination of these measured to get a better picture of how young you still are.

Keep Your Blood Glucose and Cholesterol Levels Normal. Similarly, you can get your fasting blood glucose and cholesterol levels measured at the next visit to your doctor's office. A normal blood glucose reading after fasting overnight (or going at least eight hours without eating) is between 70 mg/dL and 99 mg/dL; if yours is between 100 and 125, you technically have prediabetes, and higher than 125 is a diagnosis of diabetes. Having higher than normal elevations in your glucose levels (either fasting or after meals) tends to make your blood vessels age more rapidly for a number of reasons, so staying in a normal range makes them biologically younger. As for blood cholesterol, lower total values generally give you a better chance of avoiding coronary or other blood vessel disease. But to really know your risk, find out the subfractions of the different types of cholesterol (discussed in more detail in Step 6), because some are beneficial, while others are more harmful.

Improve Your Aerobic Capacity and Muscle Strength. You can get an exercise stress test done that measures your maximal aerobic capacity, known as maximum oxygen consumption testing. This test may be one of the best ways to measure your biological age, as it examines the integrated function of your heart, lungs, blood vessels, and muscles all in one test. Such testing is usually done either by cardiologists to diagnose heart problems or by exercise physiologists (such as Dr. Sheri) to find out how fit and young your cardiovascular system is. In general, the higher your maximal aerobic capacity, the younger you are staying. Fortunately, you can improve your aerobic capacity on your own with an exercise training program, as outlined in Step 2.

Along the same vein, you can also get an exercise professional to measure your hand grip strength with a special dynamometer. Declining strength on this test is indicative of a loss of muscle mass throughout your body and a higher biological age. The good news is that an overall resistance training program can improve your grip strength, along with the strength of other muscles throughout your body, thus slowing or preventing biological aging associated with loss of muscle (more on this effect in Step 5).

Breathe Easier. Your breathing capacity is an excellent measure of how strong your ventilatory muscles still are and how compliant your lungs remain. Two simple measures taken by your doctor can diagnose problems that can increase your rate of aging. The first is the maximum amount of air you can breathe out quickly, which is known as your forced expiratory volume in one second, with the second measure being the total amount of air you can breathe in and out (your forced vital capacity). Diseases like emphysema can severely limit your breathing ability and increase your biological age. If you currently smoke, the best thing you can do to slow your lungs' more rapid rate of aging is to stop smoking.

Stack Your Bones with Minerals. Changes in bone mineral density (see Step 8), together with arthritis and osteophytes (bone spurs), have additionally been a good biomarker that can be determined from a simple hand x-ray or dual-energy x-ray absorptiometry (DXA) bone mineral density scan. If your bone minerals are lower than expected for your age, you can positively affect them through dietary changes (such as more calcium, discussed in Step

1), exercise training (Step 2), and hormone therapies including estrogen replacement and vitamin D (Step 3).

Pinch Your Skin. Some of the remaining markers are either trickier to interpret or harder to measure. For example, to test your skin's elasticity, pinch up the skin on the back of one hand between your thumb and forefinger of your other hand. Let go and watch how quickly your skin returns to its normal shape. Compare your skin's response to that of your kids or grandkids, and you'll be able to see that they're biologically younger—their skin snaps back into place faster than yours. Of course, this measure is completely subjective and can be greatly affected by everyday things, such as how well hydrated you are. Dehydrated skin stays pinched longer than when it's fully hydrated, regardless of your age.

Test Your Mental Function. How well you function mentally, your "cognitive performance," can be measured with various tests, including ones to detect mild cognitive changes and dementia. But almost all of them must be administered to you by a mental health or other professional. The state of your mind is often reflective of similar changes in the rest of your body; accordingly, exercising your body generally also improves the healthiness of your mental processes. In lieu of searching out whether you're demented yet, we suggest that you better use your time by doing mental exercises (found in Step 4) that can improve your mental functioning and your memory, as well as keep your mind sharp for longer.

Be Less Inflammatory. You can ask your doctor to test your blood for various markers of systemic inflammation. When certain compounds in blood are present, your blood vessels may function less effectively. Over time, such changes can result in permanent injury, plaque formation in arteries, and heart attacks or strokes. Scientists are learning more every day about what the various markers do or indicate. At this point, it's still an inexact science and not one that is worth spending your money on testing, since interpreting their various levels would be guesswork at best.

React More Quickly. Finally, your reaction time, which is a measure of how quickly you respond to stimuli, can be measured with special testing equipment, but your doctor is unlikely to have it in his or her office. Generally speaking, your ability to react quickly reflects how well your nerves conduct their messages, and the faster they go, the younger you likely are, biologically speaking.

Other Predictors of Your Longevity and Current Biological Age

A study conducted in England concluded that your birth weight predicts your hand grip strength at seventy years of age, which suggests a greater longevity when it is higher. Of course, you have no control over something like your birth weight, which can be heavily affected by your mother's behavior while she was pregnant with you. Whether she smoked, drank, or had regular prenatal checkups may play a role in determining your eventual longevity, but these are by no means the only factors. You can always work on improving your own grip strength and other strength measures with appropriate exercises (discussed in Step 2).

Finally, although it's admittedly difficult to get a firm fix on your actual biological age, for fun, you can answer questions that ask about a hundred different health factors—including cholesterol levels, blood pressure, medications used, vitamins taken, daily nutrition, exercise habits, health history, social networks, daily stressors, and more—using a free online test available at realage. com. We can't attest to the validity of their "Real Age Test," but it does cover most of the factors that affect how young your body can remain. Taking their test may point out some additional places where you can improve your lifestyle to optimize your health and current biological age.

The Time to Start Is Now

It's never too late to get started on our program, and you're sure to reap some of its benefits as soon as you begin. Most of the healthy lifestyle changes and medical interventions that you can implement to vastly increase your likelihood of staying and feeling young for longer are not nearly as radical as you may think. For instance, implementing some of the dietary advice in Step 1 will already begin to lower your risk of certain types of cancer and heart disease and raise your mind's sharpness, even before you read about preventing those health problems in later chapters. Adding just a little activity to your daily routine can have major benefits, and experts suggest that even fifteen to thirty minutes of walking each day is probably enough to gain substantial health benefits. In fact, the risk of prostate cancer in men is vastly lower in anyone who exercises regularly and has regular medical exams.

So read on to start the ten-step program that will change the rest of your life for the better. Since it's a journey that involves good eating (including dark chocolate), drinking wine, socializing, and exercises that anyone can do, it'll be more fun than you ever thought it could be. What do you have to lose? It's time to be proactive about living well and feeling better for the rest of your life, regardless of your current chronological age!

Consume Fish, Alcohol, and More

"Stay busy, get plenty of exercise, and don't drink too much. Then again, don't drink too little."
—*Herman "Jack Rabbit" Smith-Johannsen (1875–1987)*

"Fish are supposed to be brain food, and yet people eat it on Friday and then do the silliest things over the weekend."
—*Anonymous*

In this crazed world of fad diets and nutritional trends, how can you really be certain you are getting all of the nutrients that you need from your diet? The answer is that you have to start by increasing your nutritional IQ. Everyone has to eat to survive, so there is no getting around this step. Your pathway to optimal health and youthful vigor via nutrition may differ from someone else's, depending on your individual preferences and the foods available to you. Moreover, an emerging field of nutrigenomics is now starting to characterize how your unique genes interact with the foods you eat.

Poor nutrition can make you more vulnerable to illnesses and their health complications. Good nutrition, on the other hand, can lower your risk for heart disease, cancer, diabetes, osteoporosis, and a number of other chronic health conditions. It can also help you do a better job of controlling any health problems you may

Nutritional Guidelines for Good Health and Longevity

- **Improve the heart-healthiness of your diet.** Both French fare and a Mediterranean diet offer distinct health benefits. Particularly, the latter diet with its high content of olive oil, fish, and red wine is heart healthy.
- **Eat fish at least four times per week.** An increased intake of essential omega-3 fats may reduce your risk of heart disease, memory loss, and other health problems. Good types of omega-3-rich fish include salmon, mackerel, sardines, and herring. (If you can't or won't eat fish, consider using fish oil supplements.)
- **Drink alcohol in moderation.** One to two alcoholic drinks per day appear to be more beneficial than none, but don't drink in excess of this amount.
- **Eat at least three to five vegetables and two to three fruits a day.** Choose colorful fresh or frozen produce, and eat whole fruits rather than drinking juices that lack fiber.
- **Increase fiber-rich foods in your diet.** Fiber lowers blood sugar levels and cholesterol. Good sources include berries, dried beans, prunes, whole wheat bread, brown rice, bran, fruit, vegetables, and nuts.
- **Drink plenty of liquids.** Try to drink at least four to six glasses of liquid each day, and eat foods with higher water content, like melons and vegetables.
- **Spice up your foods.** Onions, turmeric, black pepper, cinnamon, ginger, thyme, cumin, oregano, basil, sage, curry, and garlic all have positive effects on health.
- **Eat more yogurt.** The probiotic effect of yogurt with live cultures may improve your health by preventing illness and limiting inflammation.
- **Consider using select herbal or other remedies.** A limited number of herbal preparations may be effective in treating specific problems, such as ginger for vertigo and alpha-lipoic acid for diabetic neuropathy and possibly memory loss.

develop. This step will also lead you down a path to healthier eating, including teaching you the importance of adequate intake of fish and moderate intake of alcohol for staying younger for longer, along with how to eat the right foods to get all the nutrients your body needs at any age.

The "French Paradox": More Saturated Fat, Better Heart Health

Have you ever heard of the "French paradox"? If you saw a recent, bestselling diet book called *French Women Don't Get Fat*, then you know about this paradox indirectly. It comes down to this: French people consume about fifteen more grams of total fat daily; yet on the whole, they are less overweight than Americans. What's more, the French have a relatively low incidence of coronary heart disease, despite their diet being rich in the kind of saturated fats found in meat and cheese that we usually warn people to eat less of. Paradoxically, the average French person eats about one-third more fat from animal sources daily compared with the average American. A typical French diet consists of more butter, cheese, and pork, all of which are laden with lots of "heart unhealthy" saturated fats. The rest of the fat in the American fare comes from vegetable oils, particularly soybean oil.

Exactly how is it that American males have almost three times the incidence of heart disease compared to their French peers, despite a supposedly "better" dietary fat intake? Obviously, figuring out the best foods to eat is more complex than originally believed. It may turn out that trans fats (formed through manufacturing practices to solidify liquid oils) contribute more to heart problems than saturated fats. Americans have traditionally been eating a lot of hidden trans fats until just recently when manufacturers had to start listing trans fats on food labels. Eating less of both trans and saturated fats is still a widely accepted recommendation for enhanced heart health.

Alternately, many have suggested that France's high red wine consumption is a primary factor for their superior cardiac health. 19

Although this speculation has resulted in a recent surge in North American demand for red wines, the actual medical causes of the French paradox are still not entirely clear. Another possible beneficial factor may be the smaller portion sizes in the French diet compared to a typical American one, resulting in fewer overweight French inhabitants. Until we know more about the physiology behind these observations, we still suggest that you eat and drink more like the French, particularly with regard to eating smaller portions and consuming moderate amounts of wine.

Action Steps for Better Health Tip #5

Whether or not French women actually get fat, a typical French diet appears to be more heart healthy than an American one. Feel free to drink moderate amounts of red wine, but particularly limit your intake of trans fats, which are found mostly in baked goods and highly processed foods.

Healthy Eating Mediterranean Style

Another diet with much fanfare is the Mediterranean diet eaten by inhabitants of the countries of the Mediterranean basin, particularly southern Italy, southern France (accounting for only a small portion of the French people), Greece, Cyprus, Portugal, and Spain. Their diets are high in fruits and vegetables, bread and other grains (e.g., pasta), olive oil, and fish, making it generally low in saturated and high in monounsaturated fats (found in olive oil), healthy omega-3 fats (found in fish), and dietary fiber. In that area of the world, olive oil is used in preference to margarine and other oils. People in the Mediterranean region also consume red wine regularly, but almost always in moderate quantities and usually with their meals.

Like the French diet, the Mediterranean version is also a paradox. Mediterranean inhabitants consume relatively high amounts of fat (but mostly olive oil, not saturated fats like the French) and lots of oily fish; however, they also experience far lower rates of heart problems than fat-conscious Americans. High in essential fats, olive oil has been demonstrated to lower cholesterol levels in the blood, and people who eat extra calories in the form of this oil appear to gain very little, if any, excess weight from it. Once again, the flavonoids found in red wine with their powerful antioxidant properties also may be contributing to better heart health. Of course, you can't rule out that the improvements from this diet may simply come from the fact that inhabitants of the Mediterranean, and of Europe in general, rely less on cars and are far more likely than Americans to walk relatively short distances, making many Europeans more physically fit.

Action Steps for Better Health Tip #6

Try out a Mediterranean diet—rich in olive oil, fish, and red wine—today for better health. While you're at it, try to walk as much as people in Mediterranean countries do to gain all of the antiaging benefits of their lifestyle.

Eat More Baked or Grilled Fish for Better Health

Some of the longest-living people in the world are the Japanese who consume a lot of their daily calories in the form of fish (almost 7 percent). By way of comparison, Americans consume less than 1 percent of their calories as oily fish rich in omega-3 fatty acids, which are found in cold water oceans. Fish like salmon and mackerel have been associated with a wide range of potential health benefits, including better heart health, sharper mental function, enhanced ability to fight off illness, and less frequent cancer. An increased intake of the main oils in fish is actually associated with a lower risk of heart attacks, sudden death, and Alzheimer's disease, which, among other things, is associated with omega-3 fatty acid deficiencies in the brain.

Both omega-3 and omega-6 fatty acids (abundant in most vegetable oils like sunflower, safflower, and corn) are essential in your diet. The intake of omega-6 and omega-3 fatty acids was equal for early humans, but Americans today consume a ratio of ten to one (i.e., more omega-6s) because of reduced omega-3 fatty acid intake and the widespread use of vegetable oils rich in omega-6. Due to the way the body processes the two fatty acids, it's unhealthy to have their respective intakes so far out of balance. To improve your health, consider reducing your intake of omega-6s while increasing omega-3s—or simply increase the latter. If you can't tolerate fish, consider taking fish oil or omega-3 fatty acid supplements containing up to 1.8 grams of these healthy fats.

Omega-3 fats are abundant in many cold water fish (see Table 1.1 for actual contents), but these essential fats are also abundant in whole grains, seeds and nuts, leafy green vegetables, and certain oils like flaxseed, canola, and olive. If you're looking for the ones with the highest content, try flaxseed oil (which contains 8.5 grams of omega-3 fat per tablespoon), flaxseeds or linseeds (2.2 g/tbs), canola oil (1.3 g/tbs), soybean oil (0.9 g/tbs), walnuts (0.7 g/tbs), and olive oil (0.1 g/tbs).

Action Steps for Better Health Tip #7

Eat fish rich in omega-3 fats four days a week to enhance your brain, heart, and overall health, or consider taking fish oil supplements. Mercury intake should not be an issue as long as you vary your types of fish and limit your intake of long-living predator fish, such as shark, swordfish, and mackerel.

What About All the Hype over the Mercury in Fish?

Nearly all fish contain trace amounts of mercury, but fish found in areas where industrial mercury pollution is extensive can have particularly high levels. In general, however, mercury levels for most fish range from less than 0.01 parts per million (ppm) to 0.5 ppm (see Table 1.1). The U.S. Food and Drug Administration (FDA) limit for safe mercury consumption is set at 1 ppm, but only a few species of fish—long-living predator fish such as shark and swordfish—reach these levels. Certain species of very large tuna (used for steaks or sushi) can also have levels over 1 ppm, although canned varieties, including smaller species of tuna like skipjack and albacore, generally average only about 0.17 ppm. Most saltwater fish contain less than 0.3 ppm.

A debate has been raging about whether the health risks arising from mercury outweigh the health benefits gained from eat-

TABLE 1.1 Omega-3 Fatty Acid
and Mercury Concentrations in Oilier Fish

	Omega-3 Fatty Acids (g/100 g fish)	Mercury Concentration (ppm)
Tilefish (golden bass or snapper, Gulf of Mexico)	0.80	**1.45**
Shark	0.50–0.90	**0.99**
Swordfish	0.20–0.70	**0.98**
King mackerel	0.34–2.20	**0.73**
Tuna (bigeye)	0.24–1.60	**0.64**
Tuna (all species)	0.24–1.60	0.38
Bluefish	1.20	0.34
Halibut	0.40-1.0	0.26
Sablefish	1.40	0.22
Tilefish (Atlantic)	0.80	0.15
Sturgeon (Atlantic)	1.40	0.09
Trout (freshwater)	0.84–1.60	0.07
Pollock	0.46	0.06
Mullet	0.60–1.10	0.05
Flounder or sole	0.43	0.05
Herring	1.71–1.81	0.04
Anchovies	1.40	0.04
Salmon	0.68–1.83	0.01
Sardines	0.98–1.70	0.01

NOTES: Only fish with higher levels of omega-3s are included in this table, although their actual content can vary by where the fish are found. High and moderately high values for mercury levels are in bold and listed first. The FDA upper limit for mercury is 1 ppm.

ing more fish. This is why some groups advocate a lower intake of fresh fish and a greater consumption of omega-3-enriched products that come from "safer" sources like algae-derived omega-3 supplements or fish oil extracts. However, we presently don't know if fish oils are as healthy as eating the fish itself. For middle-aged and older men and for women after menopause, the benefits of eating fish far outweigh the risks within the established guidelines of the FDA and U.S. Environmental Protection Agency (EPA). Recent U.S. government advisories instead have advocated the consumption of a wide variety of fish while choosing fewer selections of fish with higher mercury contents, which is probably the best advice for all of us to follow.

Wild Versus Farm-Raised Fish: Which Is Better?

As the demand for fish has grown in recent years, millions of pounds of farm-raised fish produced each year have supplied alternate sources of tasty, nutritious fish. Farms now raise catfish, salmon, trout, tilapia, striped bass, sturgeon, and walleye. In Australia, they've started tuna "ranching," which consists of catching the fish in large nets and herding them into pens for several months of feeding.

Does farm-raised fish differ nutritionally from wild fish? Cooped-up, farm fish tend to contain two to five times more fat than their wild counterparts, although the fat in wild fish differs by season and reproductive cycles. Despite having more calories, farmed-raised fish tend to have more omega-3 fats, as long as farmers feed these fish with grains or other fish containing a higher content of these heart-healthy fats.

A Drink a Day Keeps the Doctor Away?

Research extending back as far as 1926 when Dr. Raymond Pearl published his book *Alcohol and Longevity* has demonstrated that drinking in moderation is associated with a longer life span than is either abstaining or abusing alcohol. One possible explanation is the effect of alcohol on cardiovascular disease. Moderate alcohol consumption increases your level of "good cholesterol" (HDL), clot-dissolving capacity, coronary blood flow, and insulin sensitivity while decreasing blood clotting and fibrinogen (a blood-clotting compound) and artery spasms related to stress, all of which are good for heart health. Moreover, studies have found the risk of Alzheimer's disease to be as much as 75 percent lower among drinkers, whether they drank more or less than the limits recommended by the U.S. Department of Agriculture (USDA), leading researchers to conclude that moderate alcohol consumption may be protective.

Defining a drink as one 12-ounce beer, 4 ounces of wine, 1.5 ounces of 80-proof liquor, or 1 ounce of 100-proof liquor, the U.S. National Institute on Alcohol Abuse and Alcoholism has reported that the greatest health and longevity benefits result from one to two drinks per day. In other words, moderate drinkers live longer than both abstainers and overconsumers, a finding backed by research in various other countries as well. The benefits are found in both middle-aged and older men and women, but are rapidly lost when too much alcohol is drunk on a daily basis. Make sure to limit yourself to one (for women) or two (for men) drinks a day.

Action Steps for Better Health Tip #8

Drinking moderately may enhance your longevity, with "moderation" being no more than one alcoholic drink daily for women and two for men. A drink is defined as one 12-ounce beer, 4 ounces of wine, 1.5 ounces of 80-proof liquor, or 1 ounce of 100-proof liquor.

Beer, Wine, Whiskey, and More: Which Is Best for Your Health?

The push during the last decade was to drink wine, particularly the red variety, to obtain the greatest health benefits. Recent studies on lower risk of heart disease, however, provide strong evidence that all alcoholic drinks are equivalently beneficial to cardiovascular health. Thus, it appears that a substantial portion of the benefit is from alcohol rather than other components of each type of drink. But you can't rule them out completely. For instance, red wine, especially when made from grapes grown in colder climates, offers even greater cardiovascular protection, likely due to its content of polyphenols contained in grape skin.

Resveratrol and other grape compounds like flavonoids and anthocyanins, which are also healthy compounds found in plants, have been positively linked to fighting cancer, heart disease, degenerative nerve disease, and other ailments. In reality, grapes of all colors, including lighter colored ones, bestow health benefits. Red wine has additional disease-fighting power, compared to white or blush, only because many of these healthy compounds are found in grape skins and only red wine is fermented along with the skins. Resveratrol activates receptors for melatonin, a hormone with strong antioxidant properties (more on this in Step 3). Blood clot formation is reduced, and consequently so are heart attacks. Moreover, if you are a heart attack patient or a coronary artery stent recipient consuming moderate amounts of alcohol, your artery walls will fare better than a teetotaler's, as faster healing appears to be promoted by the alcohol's anti-inflammatory effects in the body.

If You Don't Drink, Should You Start?

If you don't drink due to social or religious reasons, the benefits of moderate alcohol consumption are not large enough, however, that you should start drinking. Excessive alcohol intake bestows its own health problems, including a greater risk of high blood pressure, obesity, stroke, breast cancer, suicide, accidents, and more. Nondrinkers can use other strategies, such as regular exercise, smoking cessation, and a healthier diet, to gain protection against heart disease.

Will Alcohol Intake Make You Gain Weight?

Drinking excess calories in the form of alcohol can certainly lead you to gain fat weight, but contrary to common belief, drinking alcohol does not necessarily lead to weight gain, despite its high-calorie content of 7 calories per gram. In fact, a Mayo clinic study of 8,236 men and women found that compared to teetotalers, people who had one or two alcoholic drinks a day were about half as likely to be obese. Nevertheless, it is prudent to keep the higher calorie content of alcohol in mind. Furthermore, alcohol calories should not replace those normally coming from foods that supply your body with necessary vitamins, minerals, and other essential nutrients.

Eat Your Veggies (and More) for Optimal Nutrition

You can usually get all the essential vitamins and minerals (i.e., micronutrients) that your body needs to function optimally through a healthy and varied diet (see Tables 1.2 and 1.3 later in this chapter). For example, the B vitamins are necessary for the body to effectively process carbohydrates in your diet as well as proteins, and some of them even assist in the production of red blood cells to carry oxygen. In general, consuming a wide variety of vegetables and fruits in sufficient quantities (i.e., a bare minimum of five a day, but likely much more) is a smart practice. Focus on dark green, leafy vegetables (e.g., lettuces, kale, broccoli, spinach), orange-yellow varieties (such as sweet potatoes, pumpkin, carrots, squashes), and tomatoes for optimal nutrition. Eat them raw, lightly steamed, baked, or microwaved to preserve their nutrient content, because boiling them leeches out important micronutrients into the water. The other surefire plant-based foods to include regularly are legumes (e.g., black, navy, kidney, and garbanzo beans and lentils), whole grains, fruits of all colors, and a wide variety of nuts.

Harness the Power of Phytonutrients and Natural Antioxidants in Plants

In addition to containing many vitamins and minerals (including iron and calcium), plants also contain special compounds called

27

phytochemicals, or phytonutrients. There are so many of these compounds that scientists still haven't identified all of them or their exact health benefits. Some, like lutein found in cooked tomato products (like sauce and paste), lower the risk of prostate cancer in men. Phytonutrients found in onions lower your risk of heart attacks and strokes. These compounds appear to work best synergistically, meaning that consuming them together naturally in foods is preferable.

The human body constantly produces unstable molecules called oxidants, also known as free radicals. To become stable, oxidants borrow electrons from other nearby molecules. In the process, oxidants can cause damage to cell proteins and genetic materials (DNA and RNA), leaving cells vulnerable to cancer and inflammation. A large number of phytonutrients have antioxidant qualities, so they help prevent oxidative damage in your body that can cause long-term illness. Flavonoids with potent antioxidant properties are found abundantly in cocoa beans, red wine, tea, cranberries, peanuts, strawberries, apples, and many other fruits and vegetables. For example, sweet potatoes are packed so full of antioxidants that they rank number one among vegetables; blueberries win as the fruit with the biggest antioxidant punch.

Action Steps for Better Health Tip #9

Eat plenty of dark green, leafy vegetables, legumes, whole grains, and nuts to prevent vitamin and mineral deficiencies and to fill your body with healthy phytonutrients. Antioxidants that protect against premature aging are also abundant in dark chocolate, tea, blueberries, cranberries, sweet potatoes, and many other fruits and vegetables.

Eat More Dark Chocolate. Of note, flavonols in chocolate and cocoa have been shown to prevent fatlike substances in the bloodstream from oxidizing and clogging the arteries, acting similarly to low-dose aspirin in promoting healthy blood flow and a lesser risk of strokes and heart attacks. A typical cup of hot cocoa (with two tablespoons of pure cocoa powder) contains twice the flavonols as red wine, two to three times more than green tea, and five times as much as black tea. Given that Dr. Sheri is a "chocoholic" herself, she would much rather eat dark chocolate (in moderation, of course) or drink hot cocoa for her heart health than take an aspirin.

Tea's Antioxidant Qualities. Water aside, tea is the most common drink worldwide, so it's fortuitous that it carries with it a lower risk of colon and rectal cancers and heart disease. Teas are full of antioxidants, even though they have a lesser amount than cocoa. Both green and black varieties contain a phytonutrient called catechin, but green tea contains more antioxidants than black due to differences in their processing. Black tea is produced by allowing the tea leaves to ferment and oxidize, but the green variety is less processed and unoxidized. Steep your tea for at least five minutes in hot water to fully release its catechins. Don't rely on instant iced tea, though, as it contains only negligible amounts of these antioxidants.

Alpha-Lipoic Acid: The Super-Antioxidant? Alpha-lipoic acid is a strong, free-radical scavenger that has clearly been identified as the most effective natural treatment for diabetic neuropathy (nerve damage), and it may also reverse memory dysfunction in people with Alzheimer's disease. For these and other reasons, Dr. John recommends that anyone having memory problems consider taking 600 mg of this supplement daily. If you'd rather get it naturally (albeit in a lower dose), try to consume more of the vegetables that contain larger amounts of it, such as spinach (raw or cooked), broccoli, tomatoes, potatoes, green peas, and brussels sprouts. It remains uncertain whether alpha-lipoic acid should also be taken in an attempt to slow down or reverse the aging process. Controlled research trials are necessary to prove whether this compound is truly an important antiaging drug or merely a powerful placebo.

Prevent Nutritional Deficiencies in Your Diet

Micronutrient deficiencies can occur at any age when the diet is inadequate or the body's absorption of them is limited (which can worsen over time). Fad diets are seldom nutritionally sound, and other aberrancies in your eating patterns can contribute to suboptimal nutrition. If you are eating small quantities and a less varied diet, you're at risk for deficiencies. Moreover, eating fewer than 1,200 calories per day is probably not sufficient to meet all of your nutritional needs, unless you are very careful with your food selections. Getting older affects how well your body absorbs and uses certain nutrients in food, such as calcium, and your nutritional needs at your current age are likely different than they were a decade ago, regardless of how young or old you are. Being aware of how to take in adequate nutrients for optimal health regardless of your age is a strong step in the right direction.

The importance of having adequate vitamins and minerals in your diet can't be overstated. By way of example, vitamin D deficiencies are now considered to be widespread, a consequence of the excessive use of sunscreens to block ultraviolet (UV) rays in sunlight and of more time spent indoors in general. A lack of this vitamin has been linked to everything from the development of brittle bones to diabetes and certain types of cancer. The following section gives recommendations for increasing your vitamin D intake to optimal levels, and food sources for this vitamin and others can be found in Table 1.2.

Take In Plenty of Iron, Calcium, Vitamin D, and Other Minerals

Premenopausal women in particular need to take in greater amounts of iron (15 mg/day) to prevent iron deficiency and anemia, both of which can affect your body's ability to function normally. Being anemic can make you feel tired, run down, and susceptible to illness. Particularly if you eat very little meat and poultry containing the ferrous, or heme, form of iron that is more readily absorbed by your body, you may want to consider tak-

TABLE 1.2 Food Sources of Essential Vitamins

Vitamin	Food Sources
Vitamin A	As vitamin A: meat, liver, fortified dairy products, egg yolks; as beta-carotene: yellow-orange vegetables (carrots, pumpkin, squash) and dark green, leafy vegetables (DGLV), tomatoes, fruits
Vitamin D	Fortified dairy products, nuts and seeds, vegetable oils (90% usually comes from exposure to ultraviolet (UV) rays in sunlight)
Vitamin E	Vegetable oils, seeds, nuts, DGLV, margarine, tomato products, sweet potatoes, wheat germ
Thiamine (B_1)	Whole grains, legumes, sunflower seeds, pork, enriched pastas
Riboflavin (B_2)	Liver, pork, milk, yogurt, spinach, enriched cereals, mushrooms, cottage cheese
Niacin	Meat, poultry, fish, potatoes, enriched cereals
Pyridoxine (B_6)	Widely distributed in all types of foods, including liver, chicken, potatoes, sweet potatoes, bananas, fruit, DGLV
Folate	DGLV, asparagus, avocados, whole grains, legumes, beets
Vitamin B_{12}	Meat, poultry, fish, dairy products (not found in plant sources)
Vitamin C	Citrus fruits, bell peppers, peaches, strawberries, DGLV
Vitamin K	Majority comes from friendly bacteria in intestines; DGLV, cauliflower, cabbage, soybeans, canola oil

NOTE: Dark, green leafy vegetables (DGLV) include almost all lettuces (except for iceberg), spinach, broccoli, and kale, turnip, collard, and beet greens.

ing iron supplements, since plant sources of iron (mostly ferric, or nonheme, forms that are more oxidized) are less well absorbed by the body. Both your blood and your tissue levels of iron can be measured with a simple blood test.

Your bone health is also a major concern as you age. At a minimum, all women should consider taking at least a calcium and vitamin D supplement, the combination of which is critical to preventing thinning bones (osteoporosis) and fractures. Once you reach menopause, your body will require between 1,000 and 1,500 milligrams (mg) of calcium daily, which is difficult to acquire through food sources alone, especially when your diet is lacking. In addition, supplementing with at least 800 international units (IU) of vitamin D will ensure that your blood levels are greater than 30 nanograms per milliliter (ng/mL) and calcium is absorbed into the body more efficiently. (Vitamin D supplements of up to 10,000 IU are now thought to be safe for most individuals with intact kidney function.) In addition, cut back on your intake of phosphorus, which is found widely distributed in foods, but in abundance in dark-colored colas containing phosphoric acid. Your calcium intake should ideally be balanced with phosphorus (1:1), or else calcium can be pulled out of bones and cause thinning. Too much caffeine can have a similar effect, so it's best to avoid drinking caffeinated colas or too much regular coffee or teas. This does not mean avoiding herbal varieties of teas, which are caffeine-free.

As far as other minerals go, depletion of magnesium can also limit your ability to keep your blood pressure in check, and both magnesium and chromium are important for effective insulin action and blood sugar use. Selenium, found in abundance in Brazil nuts, works in concert with vitamin E to limit oxidative damage in the body. A zinc deficiency may interfere with normal release of insulin if you have type 2 diabetes as well as depress your immune system. See Table 1.3 for food sources of these essential minerals.

Action Steps for Better Health Tip #10

For optimal bone health, take in more calcium and vitamin D, while limiting your intake of phosphorus, sodium, and caffeine. In addition, consider taking a daily supplement with vitamin D (800 IU) and calcium (1,000 to 1,500 mg).

On the flip side, an excessive intake of certain minerals, such as sodium, is more of a concern than consuming too little. Eating more than recommended amounts of sodium can cause calcium loss from bones as well, which is by itself an excellent reason to cut back. Although only about 20 percent of people are "sodium sensitive" (meaning that excess sodium causes them to retain water and experience increases in blood pressure), imbalances of other

TABLE 1.3 Food Sources of Essential Minerals

Mineral	Food Sources
Consume More	
Calcium	Dairy products, dark green, leafy vegetables (DGLV), tofu, soy products, small fish with bones (sardines)
Iron	Ferrous form (better absorbed): meat, poultry, fish, seafood; ferric form: DGLV, legumes, raisins, enriched cereals
Magnesium	Widely distributed in foods, but highest in seafood, nuts, DGLV, bananas, whole grains, semisweet chocolate, legumes
Chromium	Meat, organ meats, shellfish (especially oysters), cheese, whole grains, asparagus, beer
Potassium	Fresh, whole foods like bananas, potatoes, melons, avocados, salmon, lima beans
Selenium	Brazil nuts, seafood, organ meats, grains grown in selenium-rich soil (as found in most of the United States)
Zinc	Oysters and other shellfish, meats, poultry, whole grains, dairy products, semisweet chocolate, nuts and seeds
Copper	Beef, shellfish, whole grains, baking chocolate, mushrooms, nuts and seeds, legumes, potatoes, avocados, broccoli, bananas
Limit Intake	
Sodium	All processed foods, soups, canned vegetables, lunch meat, pickles, salty snacks
Phosphorus	Colas (containing phosphoric acid)

minerals can cause you to be more reactive. Particularly in African Americans, a lack of potassium in the diet causes blood pressure to rise when greater quantities of sodium are consumed. Limit your intake of visibly salted foods, canned products, and highly processed packaged items to lower your sodium intake.

Eat Adequate Protein to Maintain Your Strength

The major building blocks of protein are amino acids. As you get older, your body may need a greater protein intake compared to when you were younger to form, maintain, and repair the body's protein structures such as muscles. For example, adults over fifty years of age may need at least 1.1 grams of protein per kilogram of body weight (1 kg equals 2.2 pounds), while younger adults minimally require 0.8 grams per kilogram. Adults who exercise regularly, regardless of the type of exercise done or their age, need more protein than this minimal amount (usually 1.1 to 1.6 g/kg).

We also now know that certain amino acid compounds are especially important for maintaining muscle strength over time. Although well established in weight lifters and other power athletes for gaining muscle mass, creatine supplements taken in combination with resistance training (described in Step 2) may increase your strength gains from the training. Similarly, it is important to consume adequate amounts of leucine, an essential amino acid for the muscles, mainly found in whey protein derived from cow's milk. Although getting these compounds through foods in your diet is still the preferred method, both can be found as dietary supplements in stores.

Eat Enough Fiber to Enhance Your Health

Dietary fiber is undoubtedly an important nutrient for lifetime health promotion and disease prevention. Most dietary fiber is found in plants and consists of nondigestible or partially digestible carbohydrates of varying types. Understanding the various forms of fiber is not nearly as important as knowing where to look for any of it. Good food sources of fiber are whole grains, bran, oats, barley, legumes (dried and canned beans), peas, root vegetables, cabbage, fruits (both in the skin and the inner parts), fruit and vegetable seeds (edible ones as on strawberries), lettuces, citrus fruits, apples, ripe bananas, and even nuts and seeds. Many manufacturers now also add fiber to products like pasta, cereals, and breads. For food labeling purposes, total fiber listed on the label is the sum of the dietary fiber plus any fiber added during manufacturing.

Having enough fiber in your diet is important because it benefits your health in various ways. First, fiber can help bind cholesterol and pull it out of the body through the small intestines (hence the claim on Quaker Oatmeal products that "oatmeal helps remove cholesterol"). Second, it also increases the bulk of fecal matter moving through the intestines, leading to greater regularity. It's not uncommon for adults to get more constipated as they age, and eating adequate amounts of fiber daily will help. Third, all types of fiber are important weapons in the fight against health problems that can keep you from reaching your maximum potential age, including heart disease, colon cancer, diabetes, obesity, and hypertension.

Action Steps for Better Health Tip #11

Eat at least 25 grams of fiber on a daily basis to stay regular and promote optimal colon and heart health. Fruits, vegetables, whole grains, legumes, and nuts are good sources of natural fiber in your diet.

How Much Fiber Do You Need?

Americans generally don't eat enough fiber for optimal health. At a minimum, you should consume at least 14 grams of fiber for every 1,000 calories you eat each day. Thus, women need at least 25 grams daily and men 38 grams before the age of fifty years. After you reach fifty, these requirements are only 21 and 30 grams for women and men, respectively, due to a generally lower calorie intake. Eating as much fiber as possible—even more than the recommended intakes—should be your daily goal no matter how young you are. The only known potential downside of eating more than 50 grams per day (besides going to the bathroom frequently) is that such a high fiber intake can interfere with the absorption of some minerals such as calcium and iron. Consider supplementing with these minerals if you consume large amounts of fiber. Make sure you also drink plenty of water or other fluids with it.

Water Is Essential to Life and Good Health

Adequate fluid intake is essential to living well and feeling your best at any age. As you grow older, you may lose some of your normal thirst sensations, putting you at risk for dehydration unless you make a conscious effort to drink more. You need to drink at least four to six glasses of fluid daily, in addition to consuming foods that contain water such as melons and most vegetables. Luckily for the coffee drinkers out there, it's only a myth that caffeinated drinks will hydrate you less well than caffeine-free ones, particularly when you've been consuming them for some time. The volume of fluid found in most drinks is more than adequate to overcome the caffeine's diuretic effect, if any is still present in habitual users, but you should probably go easy on espresso, which contains concentrated amounts of caffeine and minimal amounts of water. But keep in mind that too much caffeine can cause the bones to lose calcium, so the decaf options may be better ones for that reason alone. Make certain to increase your fluid intake when you have a fever. If you get diarrhea, try to consume fluids containing calories rather than low- or no-calorie sodas. Also, remember that adequate fluid intake is by far the best constipation cure out there.

Spice Up Your Foods with Curry and Other Spices

Curry powder is made from a plant native to south India and Indonesia that contains curcumin, the substance that gives curry spice its yellow color. Indian cuisine exclusively uses curry powder largely made of turmeric. Regardless of the type, curry is rich in antioxidants and anti-inflammatory compounds that may protect against Alzheimer's disease, among other things. An ideal way to take in curcumin, extra protein, and fiber all at the same time is to make a meal out of curried lentils.

Other spices add important phytonutrients and other micronutrients to your daily diet. For instance, black pepper contains the mineral vanadium, which can improve the action of insulin in the body and lower blood glucose levels in people with diabetes or prediabetes. Cinnamon with its bioactive phenols (a type of phytonutrient) has been shown to have similar antidiabetic effects. Ginger has been used successfully as a treatment for vertigo. Other spices such as thyme, cumin, oregano, basil, and sage contain various phytonutrients that can improve your health. So use plenty of spices when you cook your foods, and vary them. In addition, garlic acts to promote the growth of healthy bacteria in the gut.

Eat More Yogurt?

Lactobacillus acidophilus and bifido bacterium are common benign bacteria found in the human gut. They are known as probiotic, which means they promote friendly bacterial growth, because they create acids that keep bad bacteria from multiplying. These probiotic bacteria, which are the same ones used to produce yogurt, are protective against illness and damage caused by inflammation. Thus, eating yogurt with live cultures in it may be protective and another strategy to feel younger for longer. Other foods that are known for their probiotic qualities include garlic, asparagus, chicory, barley, and oatmeal.

Herbal Remedies and Complementary Medicine

Up to 90 percent of people turn to complementary medicine, including many potential "cures" using herbal compounds, to cure their ills as they get older. Usually they are seeking nontraditional remedies for low back pain, headaches, arthritis and other joint pain, insomnia, depression, and, of course, aging. It's big business, bringing in over $15 billion a year in the United States alone. Treatment modalities include diet, herbs, massage, breathing, and detoxification. Numerous herbal medicines are effective in the treatment of disease (shown in Table 1.4, on the next page) but have not necessarily become mainstream by any means.

"Natural" Doesn't Necessarily Mean "Healthy"

Although herbal and other natural products may be beneficial in some circumstances, they can have significant and sometimes unpredictable side effects. The sale of herbs for medicinal use is largely unregulated. The ingredients of some herbal preparations

TABLE 1.4 Herbal Medicines That Actually Work

Compound	Condition or Disease Affected
Valerian	Insomnia
Gingko biloba	Dementia
Feverfew (parthenolide 0.02%)	Migraine
Saint John's wort	Mild depression and sadness
Saw palmetto	Benign prostatic hypertrophy
Alpha-lipoic acid	Diabetic neuropathy
Glucosamine	Arthritis
Ginger	Vertigo

are not listed on the packaging, and even when they are, the lists may not be accurate or complete. Companies selling herbs are not even required to demonstrate the safety or efficacy of their products.

For example, certain forms of ginseng may raise blood pressure, and mugwort (Mother wort) causes dermatitis (skin inflammation). Other people have been poisoned, in some cases fatally, by taking herbal preparations containing Heliotropium when they were also taking a prescribed barbiturate. To avoid possible drug interactions, be sure your physician is aware of any herbal preparations you use.

Action Steps for Better Health Tip #12

A select few herbal supplements have been shown to work to improve health problems. However, the sale of herbal preparations is largely unregulated, and in many cases their safety and efficacy is unproven. If you use any herbs, to be on the safe side, let your physician know.

A Final Word About Step 1

Thriving at any age and feeling younger and more energetic is as much about diet as it is about adequate medical interventions and adequate exercise. If you take nothing else away from this step, take the following: if you eat a lot of fish, drink moderate amounts of alcohol, consume plenty of fruits and vegetables, eat adequate amounts of protein, and get plenty of fiber in your diet, you're likely to prevent many illnesses that can make you feel older and to possibly slow down the aging process as well. Thus, you're likely to have more energy, be more healthy, and experience an enhanced sex drive as well. So go and get started on this step with your next meal!

Exercise for the Elixir of Eternal Youth

"Lack of activity destroys the good condition of every human being, while movement and methodological physical exercise save it and preserve it."

—*Plato (427–347 B.C.)*

If exercise isn't the closest thing to an elixir of eternal youth, then we don't know what is. There remains no doubt that to feel, look, and act as young as possible—regardless of your current age—you must choose to become, or remain, physically active. In fact, being active throughout your lifetime is critical to being successful at aging well, although it's never too late to start if you're currently sedentary. Even a small effort in the direction of being more active will bring you more energy, a renewed vigor, greater strength, a better outlook on life, and even a stronger sex drive.

To gain all of the myriad health benefits of exercise, you need to participate regularly in five types of physical activities: endurance, resistance, balance, posture, and flexibility exercises. This step gives you a plan incorporating each of these activities and discusses other things you need to know about being active.

How Physical Activity Improves Your Life

Simply expending energy through any physical activity, including leisure time activities, will make you feel younger, look better, and live longer. It will even make you lose some fat while gaining more muscle, causing you to look more physically toned and younger than other people your age. An even more pressing reason to become active, though, is to reduce your risk of not feeling good during your lifetime. Inactivity, not aging, is the real reason many of us experience declines in energy and health as time passes. Studies on men and women between the ages of thirty-five and sixty have shown that simply being more physically active during leisure time keeps heart disease and other life-shortening health problems at bay. Moreover, people who are active in their forties through their sixties (the new "middle age") end up being more active and independent after they reach retirement age. Being regularly active even reduces your chances of getting colds and other viral illnesses by boosting the ability of your immune system to fight off disease. Thus, both of us believe that exercise is an eternal youth elixir when it comes to optimizing quality of life by keeping your body healthier and disease-free.

Becoming physically fit is more than worth it for numerous other reasons, many of which are listed in Table 2.1. For starters, it can greatly enhance your energy levels, reduce your risk of certain cancers (e.g., colon, prostate, and breast), help lower your blood pressure, prevent or reverse heart disease, reduce depression and anxiety, prevent thinning bones (osteoporosis), reverse prediabetes and new-onset type 2 diabetes, and dramatically lower your risk of developing diabetes, even if you have a strong family history of it. If you already have diabetes, being active can help you control your blood sugar and prevent diabetes-related health problems.

From a metabolic standpoint, it's always better to be fit, no matter what your body weight is. Exercise enhances your body's sensitivity to insulin, which usually results in better blood sugar control, as well as a lower risk of both heart disease and high blood pressure. Regular exercise can also alleviate severe arthritic symp-

TABLE 2.1 Positive Health Benefits of Physical Activity

Brain/Emotions	Enhanced feeling of well-being, improved memory, prevention of dementia, decreased brain atrophy, reduced depression, and better sleep
Metabolism/Hormones	Enhanced metabolic rate and energy levels, greater libido (sex drive), improved immune system function, more effective blood glucose use, and diabetes prevention
Heart	Prevention and possible reversal of heart disease, lower blood pressure, and stronger heart muscle
Muscles	Higher energy levels, better tone, more muscle mass (and prevention of loss over time), increased strength, endurance, flexibility, and balance, and heightened glucose storage
Bones	Greater bone mineral density and prevention of thinning, reduced symptoms of arthritis, and less likelihood of bone fractures and falls
Cancer	Reduced risk of colon, prostate, and breast cancer (and possibly others)
Longevity	Increased length of life and better health

toms that can make daily living painful. It even helps you sleep better, which is especially important since sleeping too little (e.g., only five hours a night) can increase your risk of gaining weight and getting diabetes.

Action Steps for Better Health Tip #13

Forget the drugstore remedies and special herbal supplements. Regular exercise is the real eternal youth elixir for optimizing quality of life, preventing disease, and enhancing your long-term health and overall longevity.

Exercise More, Think Better

Exercise has payoffs for the mind, too, as it can improve feelings of overall well-being, along with reducing stress and depression. Many people who feel lethargic or drained all the time are generally just out of shape. Exercising makes you feel tired while you're doing it, but its longer-lasting effect is the reverse: it enhances your overall energy levels. Likewise, movement lowers your mental stress. Just getting up from your desk and work when you're stressed out and going for a short walk can clear your mind, improve your mood, and enhance your productivity when you return to the task at hand. Studies have also shown that exercise is an effective remedy for mild to moderate depression and possibly major depressive disorder as long as the activity is continued over time.

What's more, it appears to reduce the risk of Alzheimer's and other forms of dementia that have recently begun appearing at earlier ages in many adults, even well before retirement age. For older individuals, exercise clearly improves brain function. For example, in a study of 1,740 adults over sixty-five years of age who were followed for more than six years, individuals who exercised three times a week were a third less likely to develop dementia. However, even in younger individuals, regular exercise is associated with less brain atrophy, or shrinkage, and even as little as six months of regular aerobic training can reduce your rate of brain loss.

Any activity increases blood flow and oxygen delivery to your brain and results in a reduced cell loss in the part of your brain called the hippocampus, which is the region associated with memory and spatial navigation. Not only can activity delay or prevent dementia, it may be able to restore some of what you've lost mentally. Thus you need to exercise to keep from losing your brain, but also if you've already lost some of it.

It's Never Too Late to Start

It's never too late to regain a great deal of the physical fitness you have lost through inactivity. What's more, regular exercise can improve your coordination, balance, and posture and keep them optimal over time. If you have reached forty years or more and haven't started exercising yet, now is definitely the time to begin. A recent study on exercise demonstrated that even for people who are already middle-aged, exercising more can add years to their lives, and you can be assured that those extra years are much more likely to be lived well. Frankly, remaining inactive is the most devastating thing you can do to your long-term health and lon-gevity. Alternately, becoming more active at any age is a surefire way to stay younger—or at least to look and feel that way.

Action Steps for Better Health Tip #14

It's never too late to start being more physically active for the purpose of looking and feeling younger. If you choose to remain inactive, realize that it's probably the most devastating thing you'll ever do to your long-term health and longevity.

Before you stay on that couch or in that chair and vegetate some more, think about what you really want for yourself. Do you really want to just live longer, or do you want to feel better while you're alive? Living longer, particularly if your later years are plagued by debilitating illnesses, immobility, or a loss of inde-pendence, is not necessarily a gift. Living well and feeling young enough to do whatever you want to the whole time you are alive, however, is priceless.

Do You Need to See Your Doctor First?

Depending upon your age, medical history, and current level of activity, you should consider having a medical examination before starting an exercise program. Get your blood pressure and heart rate checked, along with possibly having an exercise stress test. A stress test usually involves walking on a treadmill. The American Heart Association recommends such testing for all sedentary men over forty-five and women over fifty. In actuality, such extensive testing is likely only important if you want to start a vigorous training program that gets your heart rate up really high. If your intent is just to walk or participate in mild resistance training, such testing may not be necessary.

Certain individuals may benefit from a more extensive pre-exercise exam, particularly someone with any of the following: a history of heart problems, such as irregular heartbeats, palpita-tions, chest pain, or a heart attack; high blood pressure (controlled or uncontrolled); elevated cholesterol levels; obesity; impaired kidney function; diabetes; joint, hip, or knee problems; visual problems; a history of cigarette smoking; a close relative who died from a heart attack before age fifty; and prescription drug use, such as beta-blockers, that may affect your tolerance for exercise. Check with your doctor at your next visit to discuss any precautions that may be important for your health when exercising.

Your Exercise Plan for Better Health

You don't have to be an exercise fanatic to reap the benefits of increased physical activity. Adding just a little activity to your daily routine can have major benefits, no matter what your current age is. Even fifteen to thirty minutes of walking each day is probably enough to gain substantial health benefits, provided you increase your pulse rate to higher than one hundred beats per minute. However, our exercise plan will require you to do thirty minutes of different types of formal exercise each day, five days a week, which is still not a lot considering the positive outcomes that you'll experience from doing it, such as looking and feeling younger than your chronological age. Walking a small dog and stopping frequently every time it does its business—while a fun and necessary activity—would not be considered a formal program of exercise. On the other hand, carrying the dog and walking swiftly around the block for the requisite amount of time would be.

Action Steps for Better Health Tip #15

Our exercise plan for you to stay younger consists of five types of activities that need to be done on a rotating basis for 30 minutes a day, five days a week. These activities include endurance, resistance, balance, posture, and flexibility exercises.

As soon as you pass the age of thirty, other types of physical activity become more important as well, particularly exercises that help you maintain your balance and improve your posture. So your exercise plan will include working on five important types of activities during the week: endurance, resistance, balance, posture, and flexibility. On any one day, you can choose to focus on just one area or a combination of areas. Try to be practical with what you do; choose a few exercises instead of a long list, and vary what you do on a regular basis to get optimal benefits and to stay motivated to continue with your program.

While a block of planned exercise done regularly is undeniably important for staying younger, you also need to concentrate on increasing your daily movement doing anything, your so-called spontaneous physical activity. By doing so, you can even more dramatically improve your well-being and levels of physical and mental fitness. We will discuss the simple means by which you can increase this informal component of activity (other than dog walking) later in Step 9.

Aerobic Activities Build Your Endurance

Endurance-type activities improve your cardiovascular health, help you gain muscle, and cause you to lose body fat. An aerobic exercise is defined as any activity done continuously, increasing your heart rate and breathing for an extended period of time (i.e., more than two minutes), including dancing, swimming, bike riding, and fast walking. Although jogging and running also qualify, they are not recommended for the majority of adults over forty, as their high-impact nature may result in lower limb joint pain or injuries.

Examples of activities that range from mild to vigorous in intensity are listed in Table 2.2, on the next page. If you have been inactive for a long time, you'll need to work up gradually to doing the more intense activities. Start out with the mild to moderate activities and slowly build up to doing more. We recommend that you start by doing just five to ten minutes a day of an activity that you can easily perform and then increase the intensity of your workouts until your pulse is between 100 and 120 beats per minute. Don't be discouraged if it takes you months to go from a very long-standing sedentary lifestyle to doing some of the harder activities. As you are able, increase the time you spend doing endurance activities to fifteen and ultimately twenty minutes or more. Note that this total leaves you at least ten minutes for other types of exercise to reach your thirty-minute training goal.

Action Steps for Better Health Tip #16

Start by doing just five to ten minutes a day of an aerobic activity that you can easily perform and then gradually increase your workouts until your heart rate is between 100 and 120 beats per minute. Your goal should be at least twenty to thirty minutes most days of the week.

You should try to end up doing at least thirty minutes of total exercise on most days of the week. It is best to plan on exercising every day as you'll likely miss a couple of days a week for various and sundry reasons. So planning on doing some activity every day will more likely result in at least five days per week. Take at least one day a week off to adequately rest and let your body repair and renew itself, but try to never miss two days in a row.

TABLE 2.2 Mild, Moderate, and Vigorous Aerobic Activities

Mild	Walking slowly (2 miles per hour or slower), gardening (weeding or watering), some household chores (e.g., washing dishes), walking or kicking in a swimming pool with a buoyancy belt, standing without support, shuffle board, and golfing with a cart (But most of these are too mild to be considered a part of your actual exercise program once your fitness level increases.)
Moderate	Swimming, bicycling (outdoors), cycling on a stationary bicycle, gardening (mowing, raking, or hoeing), walking briskly on a level surface, mopping or scrubbing floors, golfing without a cart (walking and carrying your own clubs), tennis (doubles), volleyball, rowing, water aerobics or other aquatic classes, most chair exercises, and dancing
Vigorous	Climbing stairs or hills, shoveling snow, brisk bicycling up hills, digging holes, tennis (singles), swimming laps, cross-country skiing, downhill skiing, hiking, jogging or running, and most sports (e.g., soccer or basketball)

Monitoring Your Exercise Intensity

Your goal is to work your way up to an exercise level that feels somewhat hard and increases your breathing and heart rate. Your activities should not make you breathe so hard that you can't talk to someone else; if they interfere with normal conversation, then you are likely working yourself harder than necessary. These exercises also should not cause dizziness, chest pain, or excessive joint discomfort.

You can monitor the intensity of your training by your pulse (heart rate) during any activity. Measure the beats on your wrist by lightly pressing the tips of your index and middle fingers where you can feel your pulse. Count the number of pulsations you feel for a ten-second period and then multiply this number by 6 to estimate beats per minute. It is normal for your maximal pulse rate to decrease with each passing year after the age of twenty. Your expected maximal heart rate can be estimated as 208 minus 70 percent of your age. For example, if you're fifty, then your expected maximal would be 208 minus 35, or 173 beats per minute. (Note: if you are taking a beta-blocker, your heart rate at any workout intensity will likely be lower than expected.)

Exercising Safely

When you participate in any physical activity, you should include time for your muscles to warm up before you engage in more intense work, five minutes at a minimum. An example of a warm-up is slow walking before beginning brisk walking. It is equally important to repeat this easier exercise to cool down after your exercise session.

It's also important to drink fluids whenever your activity is making you sweat. If your doctor has asked you to limit your fluids, check with him or her before increasing the amount of fluid you drink while exercising. Congestive heart failure and kidney disease are examples of chronic diseases that often require fluid restriction, but also can result in greater dehydration during exercise in hotter weather. If you are exercising outdoors, dress in layers so you can remove clothes as needed, and watch out for symptoms that your body may be becoming too hot.

Exercising should not cause excessive joint pain. If you find that your knees, hips, or ankles hurt during (and possibly following) activities, you can take an adult dosage of acetaminophen (Tylenol) or ibuprofen (Advil or Motrin) half an hour before you start. If the pain persists, ask your physician to check if you have a problem that is easy to solve or to give you a stronger pain medication. As an example, some people have a leg-length discrepancy (i.e., one leg is longer than the other) easily remedied with orthotics (a built-up shoe or inserts) that will usually decrease hip and knee pain.

Finally, if you feel faint, dizzy, or nauseated, or if you experience chest pain, your body is sending you a message that you should not ignore. Stop and rest immediately, and then report your symptoms to your doctor. Table 2.3 lists some common warning signs that may occur during exercise and how you should respond.

TABLE 2.3 Warning Signs During Exercise and What to Do

Chest, left arm, or jaw pain	Stop and rest. If the pain resolves quickly, and it's the first time, contact your doctor. If it does not resolve immediately, go to the hospital, or call 911.
Difficulty breathing or shortness of breath	Rest. If breathing difficulty does not resolve, call your doctor, as it may be a sign of a heart attack. It can also result from exercise-induced asthma (use an inhaler), or your nose dripping into your nasal cavity (use a nasal steroid spray).
Dizziness	Stop and consult your doctor. This condition may mean that your blood pressure is too low during exercise. If it persists, you may be dehydrated.
Blood in urine	Rest. Contact your doctor if it persists.
Diarrhea	Decrease the amount of exercise if you get it more than once.
Muscle aches	Rest. Massage and heat the affected muscles. Decrease the amount of exercise or progress more slowly to prevent aches.
Blisters on feet	Check footwear for proper fit and cushioning, wear thicker socks, and dress blisters with adhesive bandages. If diabetic, contact a doctor or podiatrist if blisters persist.

Resistance Training Keeps Your Muscles Strong

"I am pushing sixty. That is enough exercise for me."
—*Mark Twain (1835–1910)*

Resistance, or strength, training is imperative to maintain the amount of muscle you currently have, to gain more, and to prevent loss of muscle and strength that happens to everyone to some degree over time. Muscle loss slows down your metabolism, makes it harder for you to control your body weight, increases your risk of developing diabetes, weakens your bones, and makes you look and feel older than you are. Unfortunately, once you reach about your midtwenties, you start losing muscle mass through a process called sarcopenia. Physical inactivity accelerates your loss of muscle, making the "if you don't use it, you lose it" adage especially fitting in this case. Even though aerobic training helps a little, only the muscle fibers that you recruit and use regularly will be maintained, and moderate walking and other aerobic activities simply don't bring all of your muscle fibers into play—only resistance exercises can do that. Without doing adequate amounts of resistance work, more than 80 percent of adults will have some significant level of sarcopenia by the time they reach sixty years of age and older.

What Resistance Training Can Do for You

When it comes to shrinking muscles, you can get a second chance to stop this decline. Just two months of regular resistance training can reverse two decades' worth of typical strength and muscle losses. Even very small changes in muscle size can make a big difference in strength. An increase in muscle that's not even visible to the eye can be all it takes to make you able to do things like climbing stairs and carrying groceries. Improved strength also can restore your ability to do other things that you once could. For instance, shoulder weakness is a common problem for women as they get older. By age sixty, as many as 45 percent of women may not be able to lift ten pounds, and 65 percent may not be able to lift that amount a decade later. If your muscles are that weak, you may find it hard to even bring your groceries into the house or take out the trash. The good news is that the increased strength you gain from resistance work can enable you to return to doing these and other activities with far fewer limitations.

Regardless of your current age, you will also begin to experience measurable increases in strength in as short as one to two weeks after you start moderate resistance work—from neural changes that occur before increases in muscle size. This is the kind of feedback we're all looking for when we exercise. Furthermore, major strength gains are possible even if you train as infrequently as one day a week. Strength gains are also more influenced by the intensity of your training than by your age or health status, so almost everyone can benefit. What's more, strength gains are the key to prevention of injuries, particularly from falling, which occurs more commonly with advancing age.

Strength gains can alleviate pain associated with muscle weakness, as is often the case with low back pain. Sitting is an unnatural position for your back, and if you're like the rest of us, you've probably been spending more time than ever seated. Most people experience low back pain at some point in their lives, many before they consider themselves old enough to have or deserve such discomfort. In addition to assuming a better posture, exercising more, and losing belly fat, specifically working to strengthen your lower back is the best way to prevent or alleviate your low back pain.

Action Steps for Better Health Tip #17

Resistance work keeps you able to more things that require strength. Do eight to fifteen repetitions of each exercise one to three times, and do strength exercises for all of your major muscle groups at least two nonconsecutive days a week, but preferably three.

Getting the Right Resistance Equipment

You can do many simple strengthening exercises by lifting your weight against gravity, but to do most strength exercises, you need weights or resistance of some sort. You can use the hand and ankle weights sold in sporting goods stores (starting with a small set of one-, two-, and five-pound dumbbells), or you can use things around your house, such as emptied milk jugs filled with sand or water, as well as socks filled with dried beans. Alternately, you can join a fitness center and use their equipment, or buy resistance bands, which are sold at sporting goods and other stores for under ten dollars. These bands are made out of stretchy elastic and usually come in different colors to indicate varied amounts of resistance. They're lightweight and versatile enough to be used for a number of exercises, including arm, leg, and torso exercises. Most resistance bands come with illustrated exercises, but the best way to learn how to use them is to get a DVD or join an exercise class that uses them. Or if you can afford one, hire a personal trainer for a couple of months who can show you the ins and outs of resistance workouts.

Getting Started and Training Effectively

If you've been inactive, you may have to start out using as little as one to two pounds of weight or no weight at all. Use minimal weight or resistance the first week, and then gradually build up to using more weight. It's better to err on the side of being too easy than to start out with weights that are too heavy and may cause injuries to tissues, joints, and muscles. If you're already working out regularly, you need to use heavier weights to overload your muscles enough to continue maintaining and improving your strength.

When doing a strength exercise, aim for eight to fifteen repetitions in a row. To pace yourself and maintain control at all times, count "one, two" on the way up and "one, two, three, four" on the way back. Also, breathe out during the first part of the move, and breathe in slowly throughout the second part. Never hold your breath, as it raises your blood pressure. While you're waiting for two to three minutes between your sets, you can stretch or do a different strength exercise that uses another set of muscles. Then do one to two more similar sets of the same exercise, working all of your major muscle groups at least two, nonconsecutive days a week, but preferably three.

For your training to be most effective, it should feel hard to move the weight or resistance the total number of repetitions, but you should still be able to do it. If you can't do an exercise at least eight times in a row, it's too heavy for you, and you should reduce the amount of weight. But if you can lift a weight more than fifteen times, it's too light for you, and you should increase the weight or resistance.

Doing Resistance Training Safely

Remember to breathe normally throughout all exercises: out as you push or lift, and in as you return to the start position. If you have had a hip or knee repaired or replaced, check with the doctor who did your surgery before you do lower-body exercises, particularly ones using heavy weights. Also, avoid crossing your legs, bending your hips farther than a 90-degree angle, and jerking or thrusting weights into position. Instead, use smooth, steady movements, and avoid locking the joints in your arms and legs in a straightened position.

None of the exercises you do should cause pain besides the burning sensation in working muscles at the end of an exercise. The range through which you move your arms and legs should never hurt your shoulders or your hips. Muscle soreness lasting up to a few days and slight fatigue are normal after muscle-building exercises, while sore joints and unpleasant muscle-pulling sensations aren't. The latter symptoms mean you're overdoing it, and you should consider backing off a bit to avoid really hurting yourself.

Recommended Resistance Exercises

You can do all sorts of exercises to work the same muscle groups, and your choice of which ones to do should be an individual one, based on your own preferences and potential limitations. Almost all resistance work can be done sitting instead of standing, and some exercises can be done lying down. In addition, variations of most exercises can be used.

Ideally, you should include exercises that work both your upper and lower body, as well as your core muscles in your torso. At a minimum for the arms and shoulders, double arm raises (out to the side and up over your head), biceps curl, and triceps extension exercises are important to include. For the legs, knee flexion and extension, hip flexion and extension, calf raises, and side leg raises are beneficial. Abdominal and low back exercises are also important in building core strength and in maintaining balance and good posture.

Lateral Arm Raise

For the shoulder (deltoid) muscles

Sit in a chair with your back straight. Your feet should be flat on the floor, spaced apart so that they are even with your shoulders. Hold hand weights straight down at your sides, with your palms facing inward. Lift your arms straight out sideways until they are parallel to the ground. (For an extra benefit, rotate your straight arms until your palms are facing upward, before going back to your 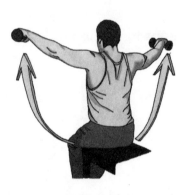 initial position.) Hold one or both positions for a second before slowly lowering your arms straight down by your sides again. As a variation, you can also (1) lift your straight arms out in front of your body (to work the front of the deltoid muscles) instead of to the sides, or (2) lean forward slightly to lift your arms straight back (working the back of the deltoid muscles).

Biceps Curl

For the upper-arm muscles on the front of your arms (biceps)

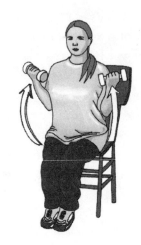

Sit in an armless chair with your back supported by the back of the chair. Your feet should be flat on the floor, spaced apart so that they are even with your shoulders. Hold hand weights with your arms straight down at your sides, palms facing inward. Lift your left hand weight toward your chest by bending your elbow. As you lift, turn your left hand so that your palm is facing your shoulder. Hold the position for one second. Slowly lower your hand to the starting position, pause, and then repeat with your right arm. Continue to alternate sides until you have reached your desired number of repetitions on each side. Alternately, you can curl both arms at the same time (pictured).

Triceps Extension

For the muscles of your upper arms on the back side (triceps)

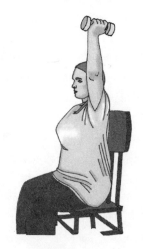

Note: If your shoulders aren't flexible enough to do this exercise, try the second daily chair exercise (i.e., chair push-ups) listed in the following section.

Sit toward the front of an armless chair with your feet flat on the floor, spaced evenly with your shoulders. Hold a weight in your left hand, and raise your left arm all the way up with your palm facing in. Support your extended left arm by reaching over and holding it just below the elbow

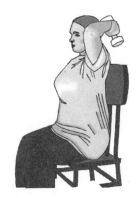

with your right hand. Slowly bend at your left elbow until the weight in your hand is even with your left shoulder. Straighten your left arm again, and hold for one second before repeating. After repeating the desired number of times, reverse positions and repeat with your right arm.

Chair Push-Ups

For the triceps and deltoid muscles

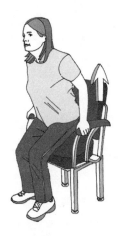

Using your arms and not your legs, grasp the arms of a chair, slowly push your body as far as you can up off the chair, hold your weight, and slowly lower yourself back down. Alternatives of this exercise are to lean slightly forward while doing the push-up motion and to push yourself all the way up to a standing position—start by sitting on a cushion or phone book if the seat is too low for you. You can also stand up and do this exercise against a wall: Face the wall, standing with your toes about a foot out from it, and place your your hands on the wall. Start with bent arms and push yourself out from the wall by straightening your elbows.

Sit-to-Stand

For the muscles in your abdomen and thighs

To do this exercise, simply sit toward the front of a stable chair and fold your arms across your chest. While keeping your back and shoulders straight, lean forward slightly and practice using only your legs to stand

57

up slowly and to sit back down. To assist you initially, place pillows on the chair behind your low back. Practicing this exercise frequently, along with chair push-ups, may assist you in rising from chairs more easily.

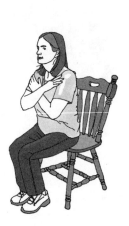 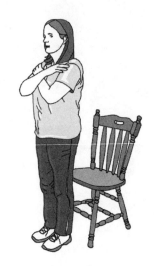

Seated Leg (Knee) Extension

For the muscles at the front of your thighs (quads) and the front of your shins

Sit in a chair with your back against it. If your feet are flat on the floor in this position, you should place a rolled-up towel or small pillow under your knees to lift them up, as only the balls of your feet should be resting on the floor. Rest your hands on your thighs or on the sides of the chair. Extend your right leg in front of you, parallel to the floor, until your knee is straight. With your right leg in this

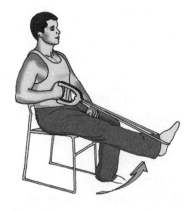

position, flex your foot so that your toes are pointing toward your head, and hold your foot in this position for one to two seconds. Lower your right leg back to the starting position, and repeat with your left leg, alternating legs until you have done all of your repetitions. Use ankle weights or a resistance band (pictured) to increase your workout.

Standing Leg (Knee) Curl
For the back of your thighs (hamstrings)

Stand straight, and hold onto a table or chair for balance or with your hands against a wall (pictured). Stand on your left foot while raising your right one off the ground, and slowly bend your right knee as far as possible until your heel lifts up behind you toward your bottom. Hold this position before slowly lowering your foot back down to the ground. Do all repetitions with your right foot before repeating with your left.

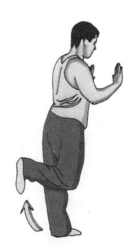

Standing Side Leg Raise
For the side of your thighs

Holding onto a table or chair or with your hands against a wall (pictured), stand with your feet slightly apart and slowly lift your right leg out to the side as far as you can (6 to 12 inches), keeping your back and knees straight throughout the exercise. Hold this position, and then slowly lower your leg. Repeat the desired number of times. Switch to the other leg.

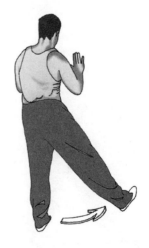

Variations on this exercise include working the front of the hips (hip flexors) by lifting your leg straight out in front of you (or bending your knee and raising it toward your chest) and working the hip extensors (gluteals, or buttocks) by slowly lifting your leg straight backward, moving only at the hip. You can also try moving your leg in small circles in both directions, moving only at the hip joint.

Squats
For the front and back of your thighs, buttocks

Stand with a dumbbell or light weight in each hand and with your feet shoulder-width apart and toes pointing slightly out to the sides. Keep your body weight over the back portion of your feet rather than over your toes; if needed, lift your arms out in front of you to shoulder height to balance yourself. Begin squatting down but stop *before* your thighs are parallel to the floor (at about a 70-degree bend), keeping your back flat and your abdominal muscles firm at all times. Hold for a few seconds before pushing up from your legs until your body is upright in the starting position. Alternately, do squats with your back against a smooth wall if needed to maintain your balance.

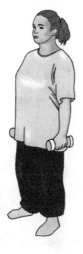
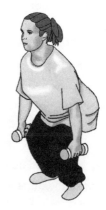

Calf Raise

For the calf and foot muscles (bottom of your feet)

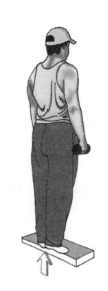

Stand straight holding onto the back of a chair or table for balance. Lift up onto your tiptoes, as high as you can, and hold the position for a second. Lower yourself back down until your feet are flat on the ground. Add in the recommended modifications to further improve your balance, starting first with holding on with one hand, then one fingertip, then no hands, and then, as you get more steady, with your eyes closed. You can also practice doing this exercise on one foot at a time. Another alternative exercise is to place the balls of your feet on a step with your heels hanging down over the next step, to extend your range of movement, holding light weights in one or both hands, if desired (pictured).

Chair Sit-Ups

For the abdominal and lower back muscles

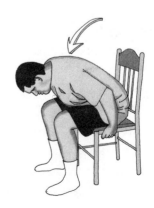

Sit up straight in a chair with your feet on the floor, hands to the sides for support. Bend forward, keeping your lower back as straight as possible, moving your chest down toward your thighs. Hold this forward position, and then slowly straighten back up. For added resistance, put a resistance band under both feet before you start, and hold one end in each hand during the movement.

61

Low Back Strengthener

For the low back muscles

Lie down on your stomach with your arms straight over your head and your chin resting on the floor between your arms. With straight arms and legs, lift both your feet and your hands as high off the floor as you can, aiming for at least 3 inches. Hold this position for ten seconds if you can, and then relax your arms and legs back onto the floor. If this exercise is too difficult at first, try lifting just your legs or arms off the floor separately—or even just one limb at a time.

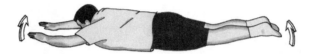

Practice Balance and Strength Exercises to Stay Steady on Your Feet

When was the last time you practiced balancing on one leg for a minute or two? Although you may not realize it, your balance begins to deteriorate starting around the age of forty. Poor balance is associated with an increase in falls and injuries such as wrist and hip fractures, even in middle-aged individuals. In studies on old rodents, researchers found that when sedentary, these animals experience deterioration in neural connections in the part of the brain that helps fine-tune movements, the cerebellum. If placed in a new environment and encouraged to walk on narrow beams, however, they regain their balance. Similar to rats, humans of any age can regain much of their ability to balance by practicing doing it.

How can you tell how good your balance is? Poor balance is readily apparent if you stand on one leg and shut your eyes. But don't try doing this without holding onto something. You may be surprised how much worse your balance is with your eyes closed. To balance effectively, you need adequate strength in your ankle and hip muscles, good feedback from the nerves in your feet to help your brain with its sense of position, and a functioning cerebellum. Most of us rely more heavily on our eyes for balance to compensate for negative changes over time in our ability to balance. Regardless of your age, if you can't stand steadily on one leg for at least fifteen seconds—with or without your eyes closed—then you definitely need to start practicing as soon as possible to improve your balance.

Action Steps for Better Health Tip #18

Poor balance is readily apparent if you stand on one leg and shut your eyes. All lower-body strength exercises work to improve balance. In addition, you can practice balancing by holding onto a table with both hands while standing on one leg at a time, with your eyes open and then with them closed. Once you're stable, slowly release one hand, followed by both, and repeat often.

Standard Balance Exercises

The ancient Chinese exercise form known as tai chi is excellent for improving balance, which is not surprising given that it's the foundation of all martial arts forms. Imagine the tae kwon do expert who, without adequate balancing skills, goes to kick his opponent and lands instead on his tush on the floor—not a pretty sight! Getting involved in tai chi or any form of martial arts training will allow you to practice your balance while gaining lower-body strength.

Lower-body resistance training also doubles as balance exercise. When you do your regular strength exercises, your balance should improve at the same time. Additionally, the easiest balance exercise is actually done by holding onto a table with both hands and standing on one leg. Once you feel stable in this position, you should slowly release one hand. This exercise needs to be done only two to three times a day on alternate feet. Within a couple of weeks or months, your balance will rapidly improve.

This easy exercise can improve your balance further if you modify it slightly. Incorporate these more advanced balance techniques as you progress: (1) hold on with only one fingertip, (2) do not hold on at all, and (3) if you are very steady on one foot, close your eyes, still without holding on. Have someone stand close by in case you ever feel unsteady, particularly when your eyes are closed.

Anytime Balance Exercises

The following exercises also improve your balance, regardless of how young and steady you may still be. You can do them almost anytime and as often as you like, as long as you have something sturdy nearby to hold onto if needed.

- **Grab a towel with your toes.** Place a towel on the floor and practice grabbing it with the toes of one foot, alternating with the other foot, while both sitting and standing.
- **Stand on a cushion.** Try using cushions or pillows of varying firmness, and stand on them with your legs alternately together and apart.
- **Stand with a changed position.** Try standing under different conditions: with your eyes open or closed, your head tilted to one side or straight, talking or silent, and your hands at your sides or out from your body.
- **Walk heel-to-toe.** Position your heel just in front of the toes of the opposite foot each time you take a step. Your heel and toes should touch or come close. At first, you may want to go along handrails or with a wall next to you.
- **Walk backward.** Try walking backward along a wall or a kitchen counter without looking back, using the wall or counter to steady yourself infrequently.

Better Posture Leads to Pain Prevention and Improved Balance

Did your parents ever make you walk around the house balancing a book on your head when you were young? Although it's not routine to do anymore, the reasoning behind this activity was

Dancing as a Method to Test Gait and Balance

Dr. John has been a longtime advocate of developing assessments that are easy to use and fun to perform, including one of his favorites to test gait and balance in his older patients. He maintains that both can easily be assessed while dancing with an older person, and dancing is more fun for everyone than administering a classical gait and balance test. At Saint Louis University, he mentally asks the following yes-or-no questions while dancing with his patients, men and women alike:

1. Does the person follow the dance steps?
2. Is there a space between the feet as he or she performs the steps?
3. Does the person lift the feet off the ground?
4. Does the person maintain balance while dancing close?
5. Does the person maintain balance during the turn?
6. Does the person turn appropriately?

Failure to perform any of these routines appropriately represents a problem with gait and balance. The larger the number of "no" responses, the greater the problem. The speed at which any of these dance steps is executed depends on the physical stamina of the patient, not the doctor. A simple circle dance with the two dancers holding hands is sufficient, but we do not recommend the tango or the limbo. However, if you can still perform such dances well, you have excellent flexibility and don't need to consider doing yoga.

valid: to establish a habit of good posture. Posture is a reflection of how you balance your body, which would fall forward if your muscles did not pull it back. You continually use your muscles reflexively to balance whenever you sit or stand. To help you keep an upright posture, you use your eyes to gauge what is level (which is why balance exercises are harder with your eyes shut), along with sensory information from your inner ears, muscles, and joints. If something affects the way you carry your body, your brain adapts and adopts new muscle and joint positions. To avoid undue pain, you may temporarily adopt a new movement pattern, such as when one of your hips hurts. As a result, you'll think that you are standing straight up even when you aren't. Muscles, ligaments, and nerves change as they adapt to alterations in your movement patterns.

Action Steps for Better Health Tip #19

To practice having better posture, stand with your back to the wall and your heels 2 inches from it. Hold your chin down onto your chest, and then with your chin tucked in, attempt to touch the wall with the back of your head.

Effects of Good Posture Versus Bad

Over time, your body tends to bend forward, moving your center of balance in the same direction, making your body unstable as you walk, and increasing your chances of falling down. Similarly, adaptive patterns of movement can increase the stress on your joints. For instance, frequently slouching puts pressure on your vertebrae, ultimately causing disks to become compressed and resulting in neck and back pain. Conversely, good posture makes you feel better. Your muscles are more limber, and you have better mobility and less tension in your neck and shoulders, back, legs, and spine. Having a good posture, therefore, is very important to preventing pain and maintaining better balance.

Improve-Your-Posture Exercise

For better posture, a single exercise done properly is best. We suggest that you stand with your back to the wall with your heels 2 inches from it. Hold your chin down onto your chest, and then with your chin tucked in, attempt to touch the wall with the back of your head. Most people over fifty years old don't succeed in doing so, but it is a good exercise to practice anyway.

Flexibility Training Makes Your Joints More Mobile

The last component of being fit, strong, balanced, poised, and more energetic is increased flexibility, which is achieved through stretching exercises. Everyone needs adequate flexibility to move well, and doing such exercises can give you more freedom of movement to do the things you need to do. If you look around you, you'll even notice your pets stretching after they get up from a nap. Unfortunately, we're all losing flexibility over time, and conditions like elevations in blood glucose levels (due to diabetes) can speed up the loss by binding to joint structures (like collagen) and causing them to become more brittle and less flexible.

It's perfectly normal to have some muscles that are tighter than others, such as your hamstring muscles in back of your legs. Regardless of where you feel tightest, working on your flexibility is important. A loss of flexibility leads to a reduced range of motion for your joints, an increased likelihood of an orthopedic injury, and a greater risk of developing a joint-related problem, such as diabetic "frozen shoulder," tendonitis (inflammation of various tendons), trigger finger, carpal tunnel syndrome, or others.

Action Steps for Better Health Tip #20

Flexibility training is best done at least two to three days per week or after any exercise session, and should include all of your major muscle groups. Holding each stretch for ten to thirty seconds is optimal.

When and How to Stretch

You should work on your flexibility a minimum of two to three days per week, but we recommend stretching after any exercise session or at any other time when your muscles start to tighten up. To stay flexible, it doesn't seem to matter when you stretch, as long as you do it, but it's usually easier to do once you've warmed up a little. If you can't exercise for some reason, still do stretching exercises. Even though they can't improve endurance or strength alone, they are important for balance and posture.

Slowly stretch into the desired position as far as you can without pain, and hold the stretch for ten to thirty seconds. Relax and then repeat, trying to stretch a little farther each time. Perform exercises that stretch all of the major muscle groups, and stretch opposing muscles groups (such as quadriceps and hamstrings in the thighs). Some examples of lower-body flexibility training are hip rotations and hamstring, quadriceps, calf, and ankle stretches. For the upper body, try shoulder and neck rotations, and bicep, tricep, deltoid, and wrist stretches.

Doing Stretching Exercises Safely and Progressing Effectively

If you have had a hip replacement, check with the doctor who did your surgery before you do any lower-body stretching exercises. Also, don't cross your legs or bend your hips past a 90-degree angle. Always warm up before stretching; do it after endurance or strength exercises, or if you are doing only stretching exercises, do a little bit of easy walking and arm-swinging first. Stretching your muscles before they are warmed up may result in injury.

While mild discomfort or a pulling sensation is normal, stretching should never cause pain, especially in your joints. If it does, you're stretching too far, and you need to immediately reduce the stretch back to a point that does not hurt. Never bounce into a stretch; make slow, steady movements instead. Jerking into position can cause muscles to tighten and can result in injury. Also, avoid locking your joints into place when you straighten them during stretches, instead always keeping a very small amount of bend in them. To progress, keep pushing yourself to stretch farther but never to the point of intense pain or discomfort.

Flexibility/Stretching Exercises

The following exercises will stretch all of the major muscle groups. In particular, focus on stretching the muscles that you have used during your activities, as well as any that may be feeling tight or stiff. Most of these exercises are better done while you are sitting, but many can be done while standing. It is recommended that they be held for ten to thirty seconds and repeated as desired three to five times.

Hamstring Stretch

For the muscles in the back of your thigh (hamstrings)

Sitting on the floor with your back straight, place your legs in a V position. Next bend your right knee and bring your foot in toward your groin area. Gently lean out over your left leg to stretch the back of your left thigh—don't worry if you can't lean very far. Repeat with the other leg.

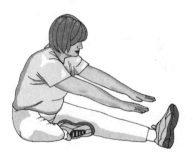

Alternate Hamstring Stretch

For the hamstrings

Stand behind a chair with your legs straight. Hold the back of the chair with both hands. Bend forward from your hips, not from your waist, keeping your entire back and shoulders straight until your upper body is parallel to the floor. Hold this position, relax, and repeat.

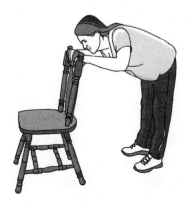

Calf Stretch

For the calf muscles (gastrocnemius and soleus)

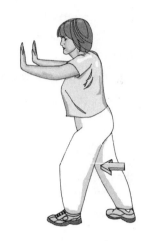

While standing, place your hands on a wall with your arms and elbows straight. Keeping your left knee slightly bent, move your right foot back one or two feet, placing your right heel and foot flat on the floor. Keep moving your right foot back until you feel a stretch in your right calf muscle. Keep your right knee straight and hold that position. With your right heel and foot still flat on the floor, bend your right knee and hold this second position. Repeat this stretch with your opposite leg.

Ankle Stretch

For the muscles in front of your shins and across the front of your ankles

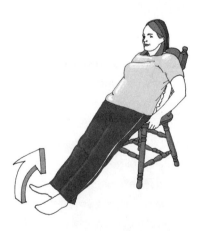

With shoes off, sit toward the front edge of a chair and lean back, using pillows to support your back. Slide your feet away from the chair and in front of you to stretch out your legs. With your heels still on the floor, point your toes away from you until you feel a stretch in the front part of your ankles. If you don't feel a stretch, lift your heels slightly off the floor while doing this exercise. Hold the position. For a different stretch, try pointing your toes to the left and the right in addition to forward, and roll your foot around at the ankle in circles going clockwise and in reverse, an exercise that will also help to improve your ability to balance well.

Quadriceps Stretch

For the muscles on top of your thighs (quads)

Holding on to a chair or the wall with your left hand, grab your right ankle with your right hand by bending at the knee, and bring your heel as close as you can toward your bottom. If that stretch is easy for you, then take it one step further by leaning forward slightly from that position and pulling your heel farther up and about 6 inches away from your bottom for maximum stretch. Repeat with the other leg.

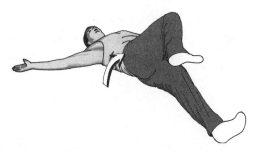

You can also do this stretch by lying on your side and stretching the leg on top. For example, lie on your left side with your hips lined up so that the right one is directly above the left. Rest your head on a pillow or on your left hand. Bend your right knee, reach back with your right hand, and hold onto your right heel. (If you can't reach your heel with your hand, loop a belt over your right foot.) Pull your foot up toward your bottom (with your hand or with the belt) until the front of your right thigh feels stretched. Hold the position. Repeat with your other leg after rolling onto your other side.

Hip Rotation

For the pelvis and inner thigh muscles

Note: Don't do this or the alternate exercise if you have had a hip replacement—unless your surgeon approves. Lie on your back and bend your right knee.

Lift and slowly lower your right knee to the left, keeping your left leg and your pelvis in place, as pictured. Hold the position before bringing your right

71

knee slowly back to place. Remember to keep your shoulders on the floor throughout. Repeat with your left leg. Alternately, you may do this exercise with both legs at the same time by gently lowering both knees to one side as far as possible without forcing them, while keeping your shoulders flush on the floor.

Neck Stretch

For the neck muscles

Stand with your feet fairly close together (or slightly farther apart if you feel unstable) and your knees very slightly bent, or sit in a chair with your back straight and your feet on the floor. Relax your shoulders, and gently bend your head toward your right shoulder. For an extra stretch, reach up with your right hand and apply a gentle pressure against the left side of your head in the direction of the stretch. Repeat on the left side. In addition, stretch your neck by tipping your head forward toward your chest and backward toward your spine.

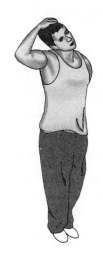

As an alternate exercise, you can lie on the floor with a phone book or other thick book under your head. Your head should not be tipped forward or backward but should be in a comfortable position. Slowly turn your head from side to side, holding the position on each side, keeping your knees bent during the stretch.

Shoulder Rotation

For the front of your shoulders (deltoids)

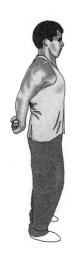

Stand with your feet hip-width apart,
bend your knees slightly, tense
your stomach muscles, and relax
your shoulders. Cross your hands
behind your back and concentrate on
bringing your shoulder blades toward
each other as far as you can (pictured).
If you prefer, you can also lie on the
floor with a pillow under your head
and your legs straight, stretching your
arms straight out to the sides. Then
bend at the elbows (keeping your
elbows on the floor) to point your
hands toward the ceiling. Let your forearms slowly roll backward toward
the floor until you feel a stretch or slight discomfort. Hold this position, and
then let your forearms roll down toward your hips until you feel a stretch in
the front of your shoulders.

Biceps Stretch

For the front of your upper arms (biceps)

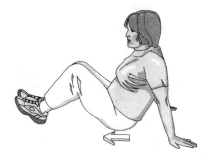

Sit on the floor with both legs
extended in front of you and your
knees bent. While keeping your
back straight, put your hands
behind you with your palms flat on
the floor and your fingers pointing
away. With your hands stationary,
move your bottom forward along
the floor until you feel the stretch
in your shoulders, and then hold it.

Triceps Stretch

For the back of your upper arms (triceps)

Sitting or standing, grab your right elbow with your left hand and push it straight up and back until the upper portion of your right arm is next to your right ear (pictured). Keep your spine and neck as straight as possible during this movement. Repeat with your left arm. If you find it easier, hold one end of a towel in your right hand. Raise your right arm, bending your elbow so that the towel drapes down your back. Keep your right 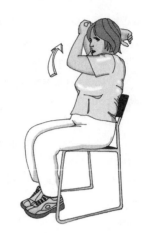 arm in this position, still holding the towel, and with your left hand, reach behind your lower back and grasp the other end of the towel. Grasp as high on the towel with your left hand as you can by inching your hand upward. Continue until your hands are as close as they can comfortably go. Reverse positions and repeat.

Wrist Stretch

For the wrist extensors

Press your hands together with elbows down. Raise your elbows as nearly parallel to the floor as possible, while keeping your hands together in a prayer position. Hold and then repeat.

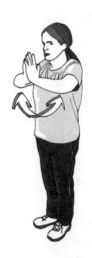

Exercise Recommendations for People with Specific Medical Conditions

Exercise benefits just about everyone, but if you have certain specific medical conditions, you should follow recommended guidelines to prevent problems. For example, if you have arthritis in your knees or hips, you should never push yourself to the point where exercise hurts, and if your joints feel sore for an hour or more after you exercise, you have probably pushed too hard. It's also best to avoid exercising joints in the same way on a daily basis.

Some general recommendations for five common conditions—exercise-induced angina, peripheral vascular disease, chronic obstructive pulmonary disease (COPD), arthritis, and diabetes mellitus—are listed in Table 2.4, on the next page. If you have another medical condition, be sure to consult your doctor before starting or increasing the intensity of your exercise program.

Can Exercise Prevent Gray Hair?

Hair typically turns gray as a result of advancing age. Pigment in the hair shaft comes from special cells at the hair root, which are genetically programmed to make a certain amount of pigment (melanin) at specific ages. At some point, these cells begin to make less and less pigment. Gray hair still has some, but not as much as red, black, or brown hair, and white hair has none. Not all of your hair responds in the same way or at the same time, resulting in a gradual graying process. Some people start graying in their thirties, but others don't until their sixties, due to genetic and environmental differences.

Action Steps for Better Health Tip #21

Exercise regularly to lower symptoms of stress, anxiety, or depression that can cause premature graying of your hair. But if you're destined to turn gray, no amount of exercise will keep it from happening.

75

TABLE 2.4 Guidelines for Exercising Safely with Common Health Problems

Exercise-induced angina (chest pain due to coronary blockage)	Alternate vigorous exercise with slow walking, perhaps in intervals of 1–2 minutes each. If cold weather makes it worse, exercise indoors. If severe, take medicine before exercising. Start exercise in a monitored setting, such as cardiac rehab or a physical therapy clinic.
Peripheral vascular disease	Start with an intermittent schedule of exercise before moving to a more regular, progressive one, to allow the body time to develop new vascular routes. Be aware of signs and symptoms of insufficient blood flow to extremities. Regular exercise should decrease calf pain. Dress warmly, and keep your hands and feet warm.
Chronic obstructive pulmonary disease (COPD)	Aerobic training (walking or stationary cycling) is best and should be done in late morning or afternoon to give lungs time to be clear of mucus. When air quality is poor, exercise indoors in a moist, warm room. Start with several short sessions of 1–5 minutes, and increase gradually.
Arthritis	Aerobic cycling and strength training may improve overall ability to function. Water aerobics are low in stress for joints. Spinal osteoarthritis may be helped by exercises that tone the abdomen and extend the spine, but avoid flexion spinal exercises.
Diabetes mellitus	Glycemic control improves from any type of exercise done regularly. Try to exercise almost daily for at least 30 minutes a day and to resistance train. Lower medication doses if you frequently experience low blood glucose levels from exercise. Autonomic nerve damage can lead to a fall in blood pressure and dizziness.

As discussed, exercise reduces mental stress, and less stress can slow the advent of graying even if it can't reverse it. For example, recent studies of mothers caring for gravely ill children show that undue emotional stress actually causes their cells to age more rapidly than normal. Conversely, regular exercise helps moderate psychological stress and anxiety and may prevent hair from turning gray prematurely. Thus it may be possible to temporarily slow down your graying with exercise. Even though you can't exercise away your gray hair, being healthy and energetic while graying is not a bad alternative.

Training, Sports Injuries, and the Master Athlete

Not long ago, Al Hanna successfully reached the southern summit of Mount Everest, the world's tallest mountain peak. But what makes his success an even greater accomplishment is that he managed this feat at sixty-nine years of age. Climbers his age are at increased risk for injuries caused by weather, including dehydration in the summer and cold exposure in the winter or at high altitudes, and they can more easily develop acute mountain sickness.

An expanding number of people older than age forty are keeping themselves in good shape; however, the aging process brings an inevitable decline in physical function, even for the Al Hannas of the world. It happens to some degree to everyone, no matter how healthy you feel or how much you exercise. For instance, even the world record in the clean and jerk power lift is 20 percent lower in men and 40 percent lower in women in the older age groups. The athletic performance of most Olympic-level athletes also peaks by the time they reach their mid-twenties, although they can continue to compete after that age. It's just important to recognize and acknowledge your physical limitations imposed by your aging, so you can optimize your health instead of harm it.

Being sedentary isn't healthy, but we can't recommend excessive exercise either. Your body changes over time, and you're likely to experience an increase in your risk of athletic injuries, particularly if you exercise a considerable amount. Marathoners and ultra-marathoners often get injured and wear their joints out more rapidly than moderate exercisers, such as average recreational runners, who don't appear to have an increased risk of joint problems from their activity. However, many master athletes (usually ones who compete in sports at ages greater than forty) spend up to a month a year unable to exercise due to injuries. Moderation in exercise is sensible, while obsessive training isn't—at any age.

Physical Changes over Time

From your midtwenties on, you'll experience slow changes in different body systems, including your heart, lungs, muscles, nervous system, and more. Being active can prevent disability from many chronic illnesses that you can avoid, but physiological aging is not entirely preventable, including decreases in maximal heart rate, amount of blood pumped by the heart, lung capacity, and maximal aerobic capacity. The result is a lower overall strength and endurance the older you get, particularly as you start to lose both muscle strength and mass. You selectively lose the "fast twitch" muscle fibers used for power and speed, and unfortunately, training can't help you get them back. In addition, loss of calcium and other minerals from bones accelerates with age, particularly in women who are postmenopause.

The good news, however, is that exercise can prevent, slow, or reverse at least some of these changes. For instance, exercise can keep breathing muscles trained and strong, enabling athletes of any age to take deeper breaths than their sedentary counterparts. You can fight the loss of faster muscle fibers by using them when you exercise—hence the recommendation to do heavier resistance training. Likewise, doing the balance exercises described in this step can help you improve your balance. Although your body's maximal ability to use oxygen during exercise typically declines a steady 1.5 percent per year, highly trained older athletes show a slower, but steady, rate of decline of only 0.5 percent. As for bone health, you can reduce the rate of mineral loss through regular exercise, particularly resistance and weight-bearing activities.

Action Steps for Better Health Tip #22

Active, but not excessive, enjoyment of a variety of sports and exercise can give you a better and a longer life. Avoiding athletic injuries in master athletes is possible with a combination of preparation, targeted training, and common sense.

Prevention of Athletic Injuries

As mentioned, if you exercise when you're older, you are more likely to injure yourself than when you were younger. On a positive note, even when accounting for increased likelihood of injury, runners of any age who exercise moderately tend to be physically better off than less active people their age. Thus, an increased risk of sports-related injuries is no reason to avoid being active, especially given that most of these problems can be prevented or treated with a combination of preparation, targeted conditioning, and common sense. With injury prevention in mind, all athletes—young and old alike—should include a careful warm-up period with stretching exercises to reduce the risk of injuries.

The master athlete, nevertheless, faces some general physical problems that make specific injuries more common. For instance, loss of flexibility caused by changes in the body's connective tissues combined with arthritis means that knees, hips, and other joints, rather than muscles, must bear greater stress during exercise. Such changes make running a particularly damaging activity for joints over time. Stretching regularly can help slow down loss of flexibility, although it can't prevent it completely, so at some point, most runners have to choose alternate activities like walking or working out on conditioning machines.

Likewise, master swimmers are more likely to experience rotator cuff tears than younger ones (even though the "master" designation starts at age twenty-five for swimming). Some strategies to lower the risk of such problems include avoiding the use of hand paddles, which increase shoulder impingement syndromes; minimizing use of swim fins, which can aggravate knee problems; and increasing swimming distances gradually.

Master cyclists are more likely to suffer from compressive or inflammatory syndromes involving nerve problems in the upper body caused by overtraining. These are largely preventable with reduced training. Using the correct seat height, wearing padded gloves, and not resting on your hands while riding can help you avoid most cycling-related overuse injuries. Urethritis, or inflammation of the urethra, and saddle-pressure sores can be helped by using a padded seat (like a gel pad) and padded cycling shorts.

Finally, not even master golfers escape an increased risk of injuries. Common golf-related overuse injuries include shoulder problems; neck, lower back, and wrist pain; and epicondylitis (golf or tennis elbow). Many of these problems can be avoided simply by appropriately warming up and stretching properly. Muscle-strengthening exercises, particularly for the back muscles, are also critical for golfers and participants in racket sports like tennis. When overuse injuries occur, rest and pain medications are helpful, along with a move to the putting green.

Reducing Stress Incontinence

Stress incontinence is when a small amount of urine is forced out of the bladder while a person is active. It occurs in women whose bladder neck has prolapsed outside the abdominal cavity, and it is particularly common in women who have gone through childbearing, even when they're still in their twenties and thirties, but it also affects older men. When you cough, sneeze, bounce, or jog with this condition (all of which are potential stressors), you will often experience increased pressure on your bladder, but not on your internal sphincter. This results in urine leakage, even if you just voided.

A simple treatment for many consists of pelvic muscle training called Kegel exercises. A side benefit of these exercises for women is that your increased vaginal muscle strength is likely to enhance your sexual pleasure, which largely depends on the training of these muscles, since they're the ones that contract during orgasms. In men, orgasms may also be enhanced and premature ejaculation prevented by Kegel exercises. For more severe cases of stress incontinence in women, topical estrogen cream, dissolving tablets, or ring insertion may also be helpful in solving problems with stress incontinence.

Action Steps for Better Health Tip #23

Kegel exercises for urinary incontinence can be done easily anywhere and anytime. Simple ones include stopping your urine flow, tightening your anal muscles, and, in women, working your vaginal muscles. Repeat these exercises fifty to one hundred times daily.

Kegel Exercises

The following Kegel exercises may feel hard to do at first, but the more often you practice them, the easier they get. Expect that it may take as long as eight weeks for substantial improvements to occur, however. For best results, contract these muscles fifty to one hundred times daily by doing as many repetitions as you can several times a day. To minimize your stress incontinence, also contract these muscles before coughing or sneezing. As mentioned, improving the strength and endurance of these muscles will likely enhance your sexual, or orgasmic, satisfaction.

- During urination, try to stop and start your urine flow. But at the end of the exercises, make sure you empty your bladder totally.
- Tighten your anal muscles as if stopping gas from coming out. Then shift muscular tightness from your rear to your front area.
- For women, tighten your vaginal muscles around two fingers inserted into your vagina or a tampon inserted halfway.

A Final Word About Step 2

The health benefits of physical activity are so innumerable that you can't afford not to be active, but if you currently are inactive, it's never too late to start. For optimal health, increased energy, and enhanced vigor, incorporate all five types of activities into your week. Work up to doing at least twenty to thirty minutes of endurance activities on most days of the week. Do resistance training two to three nonconsecutive days a week. To improve your balance, do the simple balance exercise described in this step. Improve your posture by practicing the chin tuck exercise. Finally, stretch at least three times a week to maintain or improve your flexibility. It pays extremely well to be as active as possible for staying young as long as possible.

Find the Hormonal Fountain of Youth

". . . the symptoms of old age may appear in quite young persons after changes in the ductless glands . . ."
—*Arnold Lorand in* Old Age Deferred *(1910)*

The concept of a hormonal fountain of youth is not a new one. The hormones in question are all secreted from ductless glands, such as estrogen coming from female ovaries and testosterone from male testes. For more than a century, people have been placing blame on hormonal level changes throughout adulthood—usually experienced as a diminished or more sporadic release of various hormones with advancing age—for a loss of vitality, sexual drive, and youthfulness. Undoubtedly, anyone with a deficiency of hormones, such as thyroid, growth hormone, or testosterone, at a young age often appears and acts older than would be expected for his or her chronological age.

Observations such as these have spawned the field of antiaging medicine, which is rampant with experts selling supposedly rejuvenating hormonal therapies to everyone, including people with normal levels of key hormones. Even "60 Minutes" recently aired a story about a retired radiologist who worked in a high-class medical consulting room in Las Vegas and made millions by illegally prescribing growth hormone to rejuvenate rich people. They were willing to pay his exorbitant fees to try to slow down or reverse the hands of time.

At the outset, you should realize that hormone replacement given to someone who isn't deficient makes very little difference to quality of life, muscle mass, sex drive, energy levels, or anything else. Moreover, artificially boosting hormone levels to abnormally high levels truly can be harmful. With the exception of vitamin D, which is the hormone least touted by antiaging experts but likely the most effective, the use of most other hormones is unwarranted except for treating an actual deficiency. Thus, this step provides a reality check on the progress down this very crooked path to a largely mythical hormonal fountain of youth.

How Important Is Vitamin D?

Although the majority of vitamin D is made in your skin through exposure to ultraviolet (UV) light from the sun (normally supplying about 90 percent of your daily needs), the level of this vitamin in the body becomes lower with each passing decade, even in very healthy people living an outdoor lifestyle. It has even been found to be low in many individuals taking small doses of vitamin D as part of a multivitamin pill.

Vitamin D's importance for staying younger for longer can't be overstated. The only vitamin that acts as a hormone, vitamin D's most important effect is its ability to work with calcium to enhance bone mineral deposits that strengthen bones and prevent hip and other fractures, making it a key hormone for maintenance of bone integrity. As recommended in Step 1, women older than fifty and men older than sixty should consume at least 800 international units (IU) of this vitamin daily, together with a total calcium intake of at least 1,000 mg (preferably 1,500 for postmenopausal women) every day. Even when taking 800 IU of vitamin D a day, some older individuals fail to have adequate levels of it in their bloodstream. A normal blood level of 25-hydroxy vitamin D (the precursor to the active form) is 30 nanograms per milliliter (ng/mL). Get your level measured to make sure it is at least that high, as lower levels can result in muscular weakness and increased risk of falling.

Vitamin D replacement can strengthen your bones, muscles, and body. In addition, it can improve your immune system, thus protecting you from infections, cancer, and even diabetes. Onset of both type 1 and type 2 diabetes has been linked to a deficiency of this vitamin, at least for some individuals. But avoid taking an excess of vitamin D, as doing so can lead to elevated calcium levels and result in high blood pressure, cognitive problems, and weakness. Up to about 10,000 IU may be safe for most individuals, which is impossible to get through food intake and sunlight exposure alone and hard to reach even with normal levels of supplementation.

Action Steps for Better Health Tip #24

Vitamin D is likely the most important hormone you have in your body. Take in adequate amounts in supplement form (800 IU), along with calcium (1,000 to 1,500 mg), to maintain bone health, immune function, a healthy heart, and more.

Growth Hormone: The Tarnished Fountain of Youth

Growth hormone, a natural hormone in the body that promotes muscle growth in growing children and exercising adults, is known to decline as you get older. Dr. John used to argue incessantly with others against growth hormone being a rejuvenating, antiaging drug because of its potential muscle-building effects. In line with his viewpoint, a study on mice with growth hormone deficiency showed that deficient ones live longer than their rodent counterparts with normal levels, and a later study on humans revealed that men with growth hormone on the "high-normal" side experience more heart disease and cancer and a shorter life span. Dr. John continues to argue strongly that giving older humans injections of growth hormone, if they don't have a clear deficiency, will likely do more harm than good.

Other researchers, however, have been undeterred by his arguments and have persisted in studying growth hormone replacement in older men despite evidence to the contrary. One of these researchers' first studies was published in 1990 in the *New England Journal of Medicine*, a highly respected scientific journal, and showed a small improvement in skin thickness and some increase in muscle mass, leading to great excitement and rapid dissemination by the press, who touted growth hormone as a newfound fountain of youth. This study, however, had lasted only six months. By the time the male participants in the study had received growth hormone for a year, most had developed significant and undesirable side effects, including joint pain, carpal tunnel syndrome, and breast enlargement (admittedly a side effect not desired by most males). However, these less-encouraging results from the second six months of supplementation were not accepted for publication in the same high-profile journal. Instead they appeared later in the less well-known English journal, *Clinical Endocrinology*. Unfortunately, the actual results of a full year of growth hormone use did little to deter the rampant enthusiasm of antiaging physicians from making large amounts of money by giving growth hormone to all who wish to be young again.

Subsequently, many other studies have shown that growth hormone fails to improve strength or build stronger bones in anyone older than fifty. Moreover, its long-term use has been associated with multiple side effects. Therefore, we can only conclude that *avoiding*, rather than taking, growth hormone supplements should make you live longer and improve your quality of life.

Unfounded Hope for Ghrelin?

Scientists often fail to learn from their past mistakes, as demonstrated by the story of ghrelin, a hormone produced by the top part of the stomach. This newly discovered hormone increases food intake, improves memory, and causes the release of growth hormone. At present, much enthusiasm still exists about using ghrelin to release growth hormone, with the expectation that in this case growth hormone will turn out to be the antiaging miracle that people want it to be.

In recent clinical trials, a Merck compound that works through the ghrelin receptor did not appear to be more successful than growth hormone itself, which is not saying much. Unfortunately, this discovery has not stopped numerous companies from attempting to develop ghrelin-like compounds to reverse the travails of aging. Like growth hormone, ghrelin's only real utility, if any, will be in treating malnourished older individuals with a growth hormone deficiency and a poor quality of life resulting from it. If you're hoping that ghrelin will be the one to provide you with a hormonal fountain of youth, then your wishes will most likely go unfulfilled. *consistent with premature age*

Melatonin: The Sleep Hormone

In the seventeenth century, the philosopher René Descartes thought of the pineal gland as the "third eye" and the "seat of the soul," a place where all rational thought begins. The pineal gland, which normally produces the hormone melatonin, calcifies over time. The major role of melatonin appears to be to induce sleep, but it also enhances the immune system and acts as a potent antioxidant. Although melatonin's levels peak during the night and decline during the day, the changes in the pineal gland cause blood concentrations of this hormone to generally be lower the older you get. Russel Reiter from Texas, who has spent his life studying melatonin, recently wrote a book suggesting that melatonin may be the most important antiaging hormone yet discovered, but at present these claims are unsupported by positive results from research studies.

Although it can't reverse aging as promised by some, there are some medicinal uses for melatonin supplements. For example, ramelteon (trade name Rozerem) is a drug that acts on the two melatonin receptors and is approved by the FDA for the treatment of insomnia; it reduces how long it takes to fall asleep. Currently, it appears to be the safest of the available sleeping pills and works at least as well as some of the other potentially more dangerous sleep aids. Certain individuals also take melatonin supplements specifically to lessen the effects of crossing time zones when traveling, the condition known as jet lag. It's fine if you want to take it for this purpose, but rest assured it won't make you look or feel any younger than adequate sleep will.

What About Pregnenolone?

Pregnenolone is a hormone made from cholesterol in the adrenal gland. It's the precursor for all the other gender-related hormones, such as dehydroepiandrosterone (DHEA), estrogen, and testosterone, making it in fact the true mother hormone. As such, it has been touted as yet another hormonal fountain of youth. Studies that took place during World War II showed that pregnenolone improved the accuracy of gunmen trying to shoot down planes in a simulation. It also allowed factory workers who were making bayonets to make fewer mistakes and work more quickly.

More recently, studies by Dr. John and others have shown that pregnenolone is the most potent memory enhancer ever to be discovered. Unfortunately, these findings were in mice, and the same has not been found to be true for humans. However, Dr. John's findings have not stopped a number of reporters from quoting him as saying that "pregnenolone is the most potent memory enhancer" while somehow failing to add the caveat that this finding is only in mice and not humans. While more research is underway on this hormone, its supplemental use in humans can't be recommended at this time.

DHEA: The Real Story

DHEA is a testosterone precursor that has been commonly touted by media sources misusing the result of clinical trials as the "the mother hormone" and a "true fountain of youth." Among all these hormones, its levels tend to drop off the most dramatically with each passing decade of your adult life. An amazing amount of enthusiasm still exists for DHEA as an antiaging hormone, even among academic physicians, despite evidence of its failure as a supplement in controlled research studies.

Etienne Baulieu, the French scientist who gave us the morning-after pill, was a great believer in DHEA; he was even taking it himself to attempt to slow down his own aging. To scientifically prove its wonders, he studied men and women between sixty and seventy years old who received 50 milligrams daily for one year. At the end of that time, the participants' skin was thicker (i.e., visibly less wrinkled), and women older than seventy had an increased libido, but DHEA supplements had no effect on muscle strength, muscle mass, or fat content. In 2006, the Mayo Clinic group published another major study showing no beneficial effects of DHEA supplementation. Despite all of these findings to the contrary, it remains popular as an antiaging hormone, demonstrating that humans are far more susceptible to mysticism and their hopes of staying young than to scientific process and cold, hard facts.

Estrogen: Feminine Forever?

In the 1950s, Robert Wilson's book entitled *Feminine Forever* was published. This book extolled the benefits of estrogen replacement for postmenopausal women. It was, of course, funded by the pharmaceutical company that made Premarin (an estrogen replacement pill). From then on, it was widely accepted that estrogen supplements would keep women looking and feeling young longer and prolong their lives. Numerous poorly controlled research studies bolstered this viewpoint.

The first crack in this belief came when the Heart and Estrogen/Progestin Replacement Study (HERS) was published, showing that women who were susceptible to atherosclerosis (plaque buildup in coronary arteries) experience an increase in heart attacks when taking supplemental estrogen. More recently, the extensive study known as the Women's Health Initiative (WHI) has wreaked havoc among women using hormone replacement therapies. Its supposed findings were publicly interpreted to be that taking estrogen or an estrogen-progestin combination was bad for women and might cause life-shortening diseases, such as heart disease and cancer. When the clinical trial was stopped three years early for "unacceptable risks," this message—although not exactly a data-based one—was reinforced. The national press had a field day and struck fear into the hearts of women. Estrogen phobia was born!

Unfortunately, the truth is that the WHI study was poorly designed and inappropriately analyzed. Women in it were given either Prempro (an estrogen-progestin drug) as a replacement therapy or a placebo containing no hormones at all. In women with a prior hysterectomy, Premarin (estrogen) alone was taken. The real problem was that most women in the study were already twelve to fifteen years past menopause, a time at which lack of estrogen and other female hormones may already have changed their blood vessels, making it more hazardous for them to start dosing with estrogen.

Action Steps for Better Health Tip #25

Younger women may benefit from estrogen-progestin replacement therapy for relief of severe menopausal symptoms and improved bone health for five years after menopause. However, women older than sixty should not be started on estrogen replacement therapies.

From the WHI, the researchers concluded that combined replacement therapy in postmenopausal women increased the risk of invasive breast cancer, coronary heart disease, stroke, and clot formation. This pretty frightening set of findings was offset to some extent by the report of a lower risk of hip fractures (which was the only finding that remained significant in the final analyses) and colon and uterine cancer. However, the maximum overall increased risk was only 19 per 10,000 women, a relatively small change compared to the potential benefits gained by treating severe menopausal symptoms in younger women in their forties and fifties. The only clear outcome was that it's not advisable for most women older than sixty to start hormone therapy. Thus, it would appear that this study was, in fact, much ado about nothing.

What Should a Woman Reaching Menopause Do?

For estrogen replacement alone in the WHI, heart disease appeared to decrease in women ages fifty to fifty-nine, which could be considered a home run for this therapy in younger women with menopausal symptoms. Unfortunately, due to the flaws in this study, a generation of women has been dissuaded from receiving such potentially beneficial care. As a consequence, symptomatic women have turned to unregulated "bioidenticals" that require them to play roulette with whether these compounds are inert (having only a placebo effect) or overly powerful.

Based on these facts, what should a woman reaching menopause do? If you're symptomatic and your uterus is intact, most gynecologists would recommend that you take a low dose (1 mg) or ultra-low dose (0.5 mg) estradiol or use an estradiol patch, if it effectively controls your symptoms. The recommended forms of progesterone to be used along with estrogen include a medication called Angeliq, which also has antihypertensive properties, or micronized progesterone, a natural bioidentical form. If you have no uterus, estradiol replacement alone should be used, particularly if your ovaries were removed at a young age; then this therapy should be continued only until your midfifties.

Hormone replacement therapy can be used safely for at least five years following menopause, although the exact time this therapy should stop remains uncertain. While most physicians no longer recommend its use after sixty years of age, there is not a scientific basis for this, especially if you are using estrogen alone. It is agreed, however, that women over sixty should not start hormone replacement therapy for the first time at that older age.

Should You Fuel Your Engines with Testosterone?

"O Venus, cruel mother of amorous designs, cease attempting to bring under your yoke a man now arrived at his fiftieth year, and therefore stubborn to submit to your voluptuous commands."
—*Horace (65–8 B.C.)*

The concept of a "male menopause" (known as andropause) was first recognized in an early Chinese medical text. However, it was the self-injections of a testicular extract by Charles-Édouard Brown-Séquard in the late 1880s that began to establish its mythology of youth. Based on his experiments on himself, Brown-Séquard concluded that "the question is certainly not whether the injections rejuvenate; the question is to know if one can approximate the strength of a younger person and to me that appears certain."

His concepts rapidly spread to the United States where the first human-to-human testicular transplant was carried out at the University of Chicago. The shortage of available donors of human testes led to the use of chimpanzee testicle transplants on aging rich males of Europe by one of the first "antiaging clinics" on the Italian Riviera, while goat testicle transplants became popular among Americans. In the 1930s, when testosterone was isolated from bull testicles, the field of testosterone replacement began to move from blatant quackery to a more scientific base.

It is now well accepted that testosterone levels decline at the rate of approximately 1 percent a year from thirty years of age onward. In addition, sex-hormone-binding globulin, which binds testosterone and makes it unavailable to tissues, increases as men get older. In other words, a lesser proportion of the smaller amount of testosterone still being released is actually working to stimulate muscle formation. As the symptoms of testosterone deficiency parallel those of aging, its presence has been presumed to be a cause of decreasing vitality and sexual function in males.

Action Steps for Better Health Tip #26

Testosterone replacement in men can increase libido and enhance erectile function, among other things, although presently it is recommended only for older men with low levels of active testosterone.

In support of this presumption, testosterone replacement has been shown to increase libido, enhance erectile function, and further improve erections in men already taking Viagra, Cialis, or Levitra for erectile dysfunction. It also enhances muscle mass, strength, bone mineral density, red blood cell mass (hematocrit), visual-spatial memory, blood flow to the heart after a heart attack, and quality of life in men with heart failure, all while decreasing fat mass and chest pain (angina). Conversely, low testosterone levels correlate with increased plaque formation in coronary arteries. In men with Alzheimer's disease, low testosterone levels are predictive of future disease. Interestingly, men with type 2 diabetes appear to more frequently have low levels of this hormone, so the mere presence of diabetes may be a possible warning sign for this condition. While these positive findings are potentially exciting, they are based on a limited number of subjects studied. Long-term side effects of testosterone supplementation have not been assessed, and its effects on prostate health remain unclear (although likely less deleterious than suggested).

How Do Males Know if They Need Testosterone?

At present, testosterone replacement is recommended only for symptomatic older men with low levels and activity of testosterone. Dr. John developed the Saint Louis University Androgen Deficiency in Aging Male (ADAM) Questionnaire, on the next page, to detect potential declines in levels of this hormone.

The Androgen Deficiency in Aging Male (ADAM) Questionnaire

Circle the answer that most closely matches your response.

Yes   No   1. Do you have a decrease in libido (sex drive)?

Yes   No   2. Do you have a lack of energy?

Yes   No   3. Do you have a decrease in strength, endurance, or both?

Yes   No   4. Have you lost height?

Yes   No   5. Have you noticed a decreased enjoyment of life?

Yes   No   6. Are you sad, grumpy, or both?

Yes   No   7. Are your erections less strong?

Yes   No   8. Have you noticed a recent deterioration in your ability to play sports?

Yes   No   9. Are you falling asleep after dinner?

Yes   No   10. Has there been a recent deterioration in your work performance?

If you answered yes to question 1, question 7, or any three other questions, you should go to your physician and request measurement of your total testosterone level or, better still, your active (bioavailable) testosterone level. These levels should be obtained between 8:00 and 11:00 in the morning when they're highest. You should get two values at least a week apart, and if either is low, you should consider treatment. However, also have your physician check you for depression first; testosterone replacement can't cure it, but other good treatments can. At present testosterone is only being used as a quality-of-life drug taken to improve symptoms, but if this fails to happen, stop taking it!

Treatment of Low Testosterone Levels

To be on the safe side, before starting on any form of testosterone, have your hematocrit (red blood cells) and prostate-specific antigen (PSA, see Step 7) measured and undergo a rectal exam, and make sure that sleep apnea, if you experience it, is well controlled. In the United States, men who have chosen this treatment can either use a testosterone gel (Androgel or Testim) or take injections of testosterone enanthate (200 mg) every two weeks, which you can do at home. The starting dose of either gel is 5 grams, but most males need between 7.5 and 10 grams, which means that your doctor will likely increase your dose slowly after you begin using it. Most of Dr. John's patients start on a gel, but some convert to injections for convenience. It may take three months to see the beneficial effects, such as an increase in sex drive and erectile strength. About a third of Dr. John's patients fail to notice any difference, however, and choose to stop treatment after three to six months.

In Canada, Mexico, Europe, and most of the rest of the world, oral testosterone undecanoate (Andriol Testocaps) is available, and also, a long-acting injection (Nebido) can be given every three months. Dr. John is working with Mattern Pharmaceuticals in Switzerland to develop a nasal testosterone spray. It's not yet approved by the FDA for use in the United States, but preliminary studies in men look promising for its future use. An increase in activity in the emotional center of the brain appears within sixty minutes of using the spray, and it increases sexual activity, at least in studies on monkeys.

Testosterone for Women?

"We will send women to Paris for handbags and testosterone."
    —Jan Shifren (1962–)

Dr. Jan Shifren, a Harvard physician, made the aforementioned comment during a presentation at a conference on quality of life, sexuality, and aging in December 2006 in response to news that the testosterone patch for women was approved in Europe but not in the United States. The question is, should we take her comment seriously?

Female loss of libido, or a low sex drive in women, is a common condition, claimed by some to be present in 25 to 30 percent of women at the time of menopause (in their early fifties). While it can result from partner problems, depression, and excess sex, in some females low testosterone may be playing a pivotal role. Younger women usually have some testosterone in their bodies, but levels are typically one-tenth of those found in males of a similar age. For women, testosterone levels start to decline rapidly between twenty and forty years of age and then stay lower through menopause and beyond.

Dr. Susan Davis from Melbourne, Australia, has long advocated testosterone treatment for women and not just men. Her early studies showed that testosterone not only improved libido, muscle mass, and bone mineral density but also decreased breast pain and body fat. These studies led Procter and Gamble to develop the testosterone patch (Intrinsa) for women, which at higher doses appears to improve sexual desire somewhat in women with low levels of testosterone, even those with hysterectomies. Still, both Dr. Davis and Dr. Shifren passionately believe that for some women this treatment changes their lives for the better. Both of them have spent their lives working with women with sexual dysfunction and do not turn to testosterone therapy until all other approaches have failed.

Currently, it would appear that testosterone replacement for women is at least as effective as its use for male andropause. As with men, testosterone in women is primarily intended to improve their sexual desire, and it is certainly a personal choice for each woman to make for herself. It should never be used before other treatments have been tried and failed but is probably more effective in women with true problems than referring them to *The Complete Idiot's Guide to Sensual Massage*.

So far, the U.S. FDA Advisory Panel rejected the application for Intrinsa's approval, due to insufficient evidence of its long-term safety. The European Union, however, approved it. In the meantime, many women continue to use unapproved compounded testosterone preparations from their local pharmacy or gels intended for men. Preliminary results from studies using the testosterone nasal spray that Dr. John helped develop show that it may be particularly effective in women, and its quick onset may make it the upcoming Viagra for women.

How to Enhance Your Sexuality

Has your sex life lost its appeal? Numerous studies have shown that sexuality also suffers with the passage of time during adulthood. Your sex life may have slowly declined over time for many reasons. When in your thirties, you may have just been so busy with your careers, child rearing, and other time commitments that sex was low on your list of priorities. By the time you reach your forties, if you have been with the same partner for a while, your lovemaking may have just become somewhat routine. In your fifties and beyond, physical changes can start decreasing your sexual desire and ability, but some of these changes are reversible through medical treatment and other means. For example, engaging in regular exercise can improve your sex drive not only by increasing your stamina but also by making you feel better about your physique and more desirable even with the changes your body is going through. A healthy sex drive is usually indicative of a more youthful body as well.

If you and your partner just don't seem to have the same passion for sex or each other anymore, first try to vary your routine, possibly by experimenting with doing something new in bed, to spice up your love life. (If you're embarrassed, tell your partner that you read it in a book.) Spending more nonsexual time with your partner, conversing or doing other things together, may naturally have the effect of enhancing your intimacy and your sexual encounters. If those ideas don't work, take a closer look at the main physical factors that can also lower your sexual desire, starting with hormonal changes that begin as early as your forties. As discussed, testosterone replacement may increase the desire and the ability for sex in both males and females. For women, relieving menopausal symptoms and related hormonal changes can also help. A newly

97

developed drug called bremelanotide additionally offers future hope for improving sexuality, as it was recently found to enhance enthusiasm for sex and orgasms in women.

Sometimes, enhancing your sex life and raising your sex drive can result simply from making it more comfortable, physically and psychologically. For example, in women, a dry vagina, more common after menopause, can lead to sexual pain during intercourse. The use of a vaginal lubricant (Astroglide) or vaginal estrogen may prevent this problem. Likewise, people with arthritis may need to learn how to use pillows and pain medication to allow satisfactory (and painless) sexual relations. If you're concerned about the possibility of your partner overexerting during sex, worry no more. Your chances of dying while making love are miniscule, even as you get older, which says more about how little spontaneous physical activity is actually involved in sexual relations than it does about your health!

Action Steps for Better Health Tip #27

An active sex life remains a major source of happiness for many individuals. As your body changes over time, though, you may have to take action to enhance your enjoyment of sex. Use of vaginal creams in postmenopausal women (and possibly the new drug bremelanotide) may increase their enjoyment, and men with erectile problems can benefit from the use of Viagra, Cialis, Levitra, or other treatments including testosterone replacement.

Remember that no matter what age you are, you don't need anyone's permission to continue being sexually active for as long as you want. For some, remaining sexually active is a major component of their happiness; for others, cuddling and hugging is all they need. For everyone, however, a stable, happy partnership remains a central component to living well and staying younger. A partner helps you cope with life's inevitable ups and downs and is there to help you when you need emotional support. For others, masturbation is a normal replacement for a partner who is no longer available. Consenting older adults involved in unusual sexual practices, such as sadomasochism or homosexuality, simply need to make their physician aware of their choices so that their rights to continue with less mainstream behaviors will be respected.

More than half of middle-aged men have some form of impotence, which has been renamed erectile dysfunction, or ED, for reasons of political correctness. By now, we all know that Bob Dole had it, and at one time or another so have most of our male friends and acquaintances. The most common cause of ED is blockage of the blood vessels going to the penis, which decreases blood flow there. Numerous other causes from depression to nerve problems, medication effects, and low testosterone levels exist, but cigarette smoking is the most common lifestyle choice that causes ED. Males with ED are at greater risk for heart attacks, stroke, and peripheral vascular disease, so if you have it, your physician needs to diligently search for other treatable sites of blood vessel disease in your body.

Viagra, like Xerox, has become part of our language. Today most males with ED usually are offered Viagra, Cialis, or Levitra. When Viagra and the other choices don't work and if you have low testosterone levels, replacement therapy may restore your sexual vigor and enjoyment of life. Other treatments include injections of various compounds directly into the penis and urethral suppositories that can also produce erections. For highly sexually active men, a penile prosthesis remains the best option, although it's admittedly getting more difficult to find an experienced urologist to undertake this procedure since the advent of Viagra. Some other products are also on the horizon, such as a drug called Uprima and the aforementioned bremelanotide (with regard to women), both of which can also be used to improve erectile performance in males through its direct action on the brain. Keep in mind that fixing ED will not heal clogged arteries or a troubled relationship, and the steps to be taken should be discussed with both partners before any heroic measures are tried.

A Final Word About Step 3

Hormone use in the quest for eternal youth represents a double-edged sword for all adults. While almost everyone can benefit from supplemental vitamin D, other hormonal options such as testosterone and estrogen replacement therapies should be used to treat specific symptoms at your request. Growth hormone use can be positively dangerous and is best avoided, although melatonin may help you fall asleep a little more easily. Sexuality can remain important throughout your lifetime, and a healthy sex drive during all of your adult years is a sign of a healthy body and a source of youthful vigor.

4

Stay Active
for a Sharper Mind

"Memory is a passion no less powerful or pervasive than love."
—*Elie Wiesel (1928–), in* All Rivers Run to the Sea

"There is a fountain of youth. It is your mind, your talents, the creativity you bring to your life and the lives of the people you love. When you learn to tap this resource, you will have defeated age."
—*Sophia Loren (1934–)*

The most precious resource of all human beings is our ability to reason and interact with the world around us. Luckily, healthy adults can maintain their overall intellectual performance into their eighties and beyond. Your language ability, sensory and immediate memory, and problem-solving skills normally will change little over time. An important part of staying younger, however, is taking steps to exercise your mind, including your thinking ability and your learning capacity, to keep all of your mental processes working optimally. Think of your brain as just another muscle, one that has to be exercised regularly to keep it in optimal condition. This step lets you know how to get started, by giving you specific memory exercises and ways to reverse memory loss.

It's also important to know how to distinguish between normal memory lapses and more serious mind-related problems, such as depression, dementia, mild cognitive impairment, and Alzheimer's disease, that may be treatable to enhance your enjoyment of life. Likewise, spirituality and religion are a comfort to many individuals and can provide much-needed emotional support. You should also realize that a high level of creativity is possible throughout your life span, and examples of the creative works of older minds abound. Read on to get started in keeping your mind, along with your body, in tip-top shape throughout your lifetime.

Creativity and Aging

To start on a positive note, growing older by no means results in an inevitable end to your creative thought processes. On the contrary, the concept that you can and will continue having a productive life for years to come has been demonstrated by many and has been encapsulated by poets throughout the ages, from Seneca, who stated, "The best morsel is reserved to the last," to Robert Browning, who exclaimed, "Grow old with me! The best is yet to be."

Examples abound of extraordinarily creative older people whose achievements vie with those of anyone younger. As poetically detailed by Henry Wadsworth Longfellow, "Nothing is too late till the tired heart shall cease to palpitate." Among scientists, Galileo changed our view of the earth—round versus flat—when he was a robust 74. Benjamin Franklin gave us bifocal glasses at 78, and Sigmund Freud's *The Ego and the Id* was published when he was 67. Giuseppe Verdi wrote *Otello* at 74 and *Falstaff* at 80. Richard Wagner's *Ring* operas were written after his 60th birthday. George Bernard Shaw continued to write plays into his 90s, Goethe wrote the second part of *Faust* at 80, and Cervantes was in his 60s when he wrote *Don Quixote*. Prolific author James Michener wrote ten very long books in the last 4 years of his over-90-year life.

Among artists and performers, Michelangelo produced two *Pietàs*, one at 22 and the other at 90. His *Last Judgment* was painted when he was relatively young: between 57 and 66 years old. Pablo Picasso was extraordinarily productive throughout life, Henri Matisse did his cutouts in old age, and Grandma Moses produced her last painting at age 103. Interestingly, Claude Monet did his best Impressionist art after he developed cataracts. Finally, on the big screen, actress Jessica Tandy won an Oscar for her colorful performance in *Driving Miss Daisy* in 1989 when she was 80 years of age, making her the oldest actor or actress ever to win an Academy Award, beating out George Burns by just 1 year for his work in *The Sunshine Boys* at the age of 79. When he reached the one-century mark in 1996, he had successfully spent 80 years in show business, appearing in his last movie just 2 years before his death occurring not long after his 100th birthday.

What Causes Memory Loss, and How Much Is Normal?

Whether you're still creative or not, you're likely to experience a decrease in your ability to learn and remember things as you age. For instance, a study of Harvard physicians found that between forty and seventy years of age, most of them experienced an approximate 18 percent decrease in this ability. While the extent of changes in learning ability varies widely from person to person, everyone shows some degree of decline over time, along with reductions in skills like riding a bike or judging distances accurately.

Memory loss, or not being able to remember what you've already learned, is a different ball game, but it can be a frightening occurrence whether it's minor forgetfulness or the devastating effects of Alzheimer's disease. How much memory loss is normal? Although you will experience a slower rate of learning and memorizing things, you should not lose your memory—short-term or long-term—simply from getting older. Some degree of forgetfulness is normal, but you should maintain the ability to function in your job and remember the names of your spouse, children, friends, and so on. In fact, you should never forget the names of your close relatives and friends, as forgetting who they are would be abnormal. The kind of memory loss that would be concerning is completely forgetting entire events. For example, it would be normal to not recall the name of a movie you saw last weekend, but it's not normal to forget that you saw a movie at all.

The most common causes of normal memory loss are stress and anxiety, followed by depression, all of which are considered reversible. Only after these emotional states are eliminated would other medical conditions be considered as potential causes, and Alzheimer's disease would actually be far down the list. Most older adults who complain about memory loss do not have Alzheimer's disease; rather, many are either experiencing normal forgetfulness or suffering from mild mental impairment, depression, stress, anxiety, fatigue, lack of sufficient sleep, or other medical issues (such as a prior head trauma resulting in unconsciousness) that are impacting their short-term memory.

Action Steps for Better Health Tip #28

Everyone experiences a decreased ability to learn and memorize things over time, but while some degree of forgetfulness is normal, memory loss is not usual. For instance, it would not be concerning to forget the name of a movie you saw last weekend, but you shouldn't forget that you saw a movie at all.

Before a person can be diagnosed as having Alzheimer's disease or even dementia, the reversible causes of memory loss should be treated first. These potential causes are listed in Table 4.1, along with ways to treat each problem and restore memory function. Sometimes the cure is incredibly simple, such as when medical students at Saint Louis University found that removing excess wax from the ears of nursing home residents improved their mental

TABLE 4.1 Reversing Memory Loss

Cause of Memory Loss	How to Restore Memory
Emotional states, such as depression and anxiety	Treat mild to moderate depression and anxiety with physical activity and antidepressant or antianxiety medications.
Uncontrolled metabolic disorders, such as diabetes and thyroid hormone production problems	Control blood glucose levels with diabetic medications, exercise, and diet; take synthetic thyroid hormones.
Hearing and vision problems	Use hearing aids, clean out excess earwax, and correct vision with glasses, if possible.
Drugs, including certain antidepressants, antipsychotics, digoxin, and others	Avoid taking drugs that cause lesser mental functioning and memory loss, or try taking lower doses of them.
Anemia: low hemoglobin levels, fewer red blood cells	Boost red blood cells naturally with prescription medications, such as erythropoietin or darbepoetin.
Infections such as syphilis, AIDS, Lyme disease, and many others	Treat infections with antibiotics and other appropriate medications.
Benign or malignant brain tumors	Remove tumors through surgery.

status more than most drugs did. People with uncontrolled diabetes can act impaired because blood glucose levels higher than 200 mg/dL interfere with normal learning and memory, as do triglyceride (blood fat) levels higher than 150 mg/dL. Likewise, aggressive treatment of anemia using hormones like erythropoietin to boost red blood cells improves mental function as soon as oxygen delivery to the brain is enhanced.

Exercise Your Mind to Keep It Healthy

Not surprisingly, the same advice that we gave for achieving physical fitness applies to mental fitness: "Use it or lose it." Just as daily exercise strengthens certain muscle groups, mental exercises will strengthen and enhance your cognitive function. The goal of brain fitness is to revive certain mental abilities before they slow down or reverse such changes if they have already taken place. The exercises in the sidebar titled "Mental Exercises for a Healthier

Mental Exercises for a Healthier Mind

- Try to memorize any sort of list, and at the end of the day, try to recall as many of the items as you can. You can memorize any list that is new to you (e.g., a list of groceries you need that week), but try to make it as challenging as possible for maximum mental stimulation.

- Each time you answer the phone, practice recognizing the callers before they identify themselves. Then memorize the caller's phone number. At the end of the day and later at the end of the week, try to write down the names of all the people you have spoken with and their phone numbers.

- Pick an object each day to observe and then draw (to stimulate your short-term memory). To work your long-term memory, at the end of the week draw all seven objects from each day of the week without looking to see what they were.

- Whenever you walk into a room, try to quickly determine how many people, pieces of furniture, and other objects in it are on your right and on your left. Also, pick out any details that have changed since your last visit, if it's a usual room.

- When you have visited somewhere and then return home, try to draw a plan or map of the place you have seen. Repeat this exercise every time you return from somewhere new.

- Take a sentence from something you are reading and try to make other sentences using the same words, but in a different order. As an alternative, try substituting new words in several places without making the sentence nonsensical.

- Try playing challenging card or board games that require mental reasoning, such as pinochle, bridge, chess, checkers, or Othello. To keep them fresh and challenging, avoid playing the same games all the time.

- Do daily crossword puzzles, anagrams, and other word or reasoning games. Recently, Sudoku has become an excellent source of such exercises.

- Find new games and interests, as well as different activities and partners for your chosen games and activities.
- Listen to or read the news; later on, try to write down a summary, or main points, of all that you heard or read.
- Read challenging articles and books, including nonfiction, fiction, poetry, classic literature, and more.
- When you see a word, think of as many others that begin with the same two letters as you can. Alternately, use the last two letters of the word and think of other words with that ending.
- When eating, try to identify the individual ingredients in what you're eating, including the subtle flavorings of herbs and spices. Exercise your senses of smell and touch by trying to identify objects with your eyes closed, both indoors and outdoors.
- Try to do something new or unusual every day that requires you to think. For example, vary the route that you take home to see if you can figure out a slightly different way to arrive at your usual destination.
- Practice doing math problems in your head: adding, subtracting, multiplying, figuring out percentages from decimals, and so on. Practice to get better at doing any types of math problems that you find particularly challenging.
- Learn a new language, either on your own or by taking a class. Sign up for other courses that are challenging and fun.
- Play video games, particularly ones that require quick responses. It will give you something to do with your kids, grandkids, and great-grandkids.
- Use your imagination and your creativity to think up new ways to exercise your mind on a daily basis.

Mind" are recommended to combat mental sluggishness. They focus on stimulating all of your senses, as well as logical thinking and mental reasoning.

Action Steps for Better Health Tip #29

Exercising both your mind and your body with daily exercises can keep your mental status sharper. Do daily (and varied) mental and physical activity for optimal mental sharpness and physical fitness.

Exercise Your Body for a Healthy Mind

Just as you need to exercise your mind to keep the neurons firing well and your mental processes sharp, exercising your body will also keep your mind healthy. Exercise can improve not only your physical health but also your mental well-being, because almost all forms of physical activity improve insulin sensitivity and simultaneously decrease your risk of vascular changes—one of the risk factors for dementia and cognitive declines. Participation in leisure physical activities reduces your risk, and all levels of exercise may prevent or delay the onset of dementia or Alzheimer's. If you're already suffering from some noticeable mental changes, all is not lost. Exercise training also improves mental functioning and positive behavior in people who have already developed some level of dementia and other related cognitive changes.

Exercise improves memory and mental function in two ways. First, it enhances your heart's function, which means that it can pump more effectively and perfuse your brain with a rich supply of blood, along with lowering your risk for vascular problems. Second, exercise also has a direct impact on growth factors in the brain, which are proteins that naturally nourish the brain cells and help repair small injuries, thus allowing them to remain healthy and functional. Two of these growth factors, brain-derived neurotrophic factor and nerve growth factor, have both been shown to increase with exercise and to improve memory. Thus exercise makes your brain repair itself to allow it to work better.

Regular physical activity can additionally alleviate many of the reversible causes of memory loss by reducing stress, anxiety, depression, and sleep disorders. Any type of physical activity is an effective, but often underused, treatment for mild to moderate depression and emotional stress. Exercising helps you release fewer stress hormones as well, which will help you sleep better, gain less fat weight, and keep your immune system stronger. To treat anxiety, more intense exercise may be more effective because it causes a greater release of beta-endorphins, which are brain hormones with calming effects.

Singing the Blues: Dealing with Depression

While dementia is the most common mental illness to afflict older people, depression is more devastating for the individual and family members, and it can occur at any age. Pervasive sadness can totally destroy your ability to function, often leading to suicidal thoughts and actions. In addition, living with depressed individuals can leave the rest of the family exhausted and drained of all their enthusiasm for life. Feeling blue can negatively impact all aspects of living well, both mental and physical, but the good news is that it's treatable.

Who Gets Depressed and Why?

Despite the general expectation that older people's life experiences, such as losing a spouse, job, house, or friends, lead to justifiable depression, major depressive disorders occur more commonly in young women and men than in older ones. Older people generally cope better with disease and adversity than their younger counterparts. However, as people begin to suffer from more diseases and decreased feelings of youthfulness, even older individuals may develop an intermediate version of sadness known as dysphoria. Moreover, if you become depressed when you're older, it's more likely to go unrecognized and untreated. For this reason, early detection and treatment is essential, particularly for anyone older than fifty.

Depressive symptoms are often atypical, meaning that the usual ones may not be prominent or even evident. Some people may complain about dizziness or loud tinnitus (ringing in their ears), or they may experience severe weight loss. Depression can even be misdiagnosed as dementia or cognitive impairment. When you're depressed, you often lack the desire to answer questions that may detect depression. Suicide occurs most commonly in older white males, and two out of three people who commit suicide actually will have had a doctor's appointment in the month before. They generally have no specific complaints of depression, and consequently, their cry for help is often missed. When anyone ever says that he or she is thinking of suicide, this statement must be taken seriously and appropriate treatments started right away.

A number of medical conditions are also associated with a greater risk of depression, including pancreatic cancer, stroke, Parkinson's disease, diabetes, and most hormonal disorders. The major neurotransmitter abnormalities resulting in depression are related to norepinephrine and serotonin, both of which are substances found in the brain. Elevated levels of another hormone, corticotropin-releasing factor, appears to cause most of the vegetative signs of depression, including weight loss, sleep disturbances, constipation, erectile dysfunction, and decreased libido. It's also responsible for elevating blood cortisol levels, which causes faster bone thinning and decreased insulin action. What's more, if you're depressed and have a heart attack, you're likely to fare less well and have another cardiac problem within a year.

Action Steps for Better Health Tip #30

Depression is a common and emotionally devastating condition that can strike at any age and often goes undetected and untreated the older you are. If you feel unusually sad for an extended period, seek out treatment from your physician before you end up with limitations from physical symptoms as well.

How Depression Is Treated

Depression is effectively treated with psychotherapy (talk therapy), drugs, and electroconvulsive therapy (shock therapy). One-third or more of people with depression will spontaneously get better, and drugs and psychotherapy will cure approximately another third. Electroconvulsive therapy will cure eight out of ten people, but is less commonly used.

Numerous drugs have been developed for the treatment of depression. The two major classes are tricyclics, which alter norepinephrine function, and serotonin reuptake inhibitors (SSRIs) that may be more effective for severe depression. Tricyclics are more sedative and have a large number of potentially undesirable side effects, including an increased risk of glaucoma, abnormal heart rhythms, urinary retention and incontinence, hip fractures, and falls. A large number of SSRIs are available, and although many physicians consider them to be safer to use than tricyclics, SSRIs have many potential side effects. For instance, they can cause low sodium levels in blood, stomach bleeding, hip fractures, falls, sleep disturbances, and more. Thus, neither class of drugs has potential side effects that are desirable.

In addition to traditional medical therapy, some herbal remedies for depression have been tried. For example, Saint John's wort (*hypericum perforatum*) is an herbal drug that has shown efficacy against mild (but not major) depression in some studies. It appears to have fewer side effects than tricyclics or SSRIs but has not been thoroughly studied in this regard.

Emotionally Speaking, Where Do We Go from Here?

For some reason, psychologically ill persons are often blamed for their problems. Physicians have little difficulty treating the physical ailments of smokers, alcoholics, drug abusers, obese individuals, and those with sexually transmitted diseases. Yet they often fail to prescribe appropriate therapies for emotional changes. When a mind malfunctions, one or more neurotransmitters have now started to jump in the wrong rhythm or are failing to be recognized by the receptors that normally receive them. Such a phenomenon is no different from many metabolic disorders, such as diabetes, or classical neurological disorders like epilepsy or multiple sclerosis. It's time to make treatment of major mental health disorders a central part of staying young.

What Are Mild Neurocognitive Disorder and Dementia?

Being cognitively impaired, becoming demented, or suffering from Alzheimer's disease are not possibilities that anyone wants to dwell on. Nevertheless, it's important to understand what causes such mental changes, so that if there is anything preventive that you can do, you have the option of trying to keep your mental function intact. As discussed, all individuals lose some of the ability to learn things at the rate they did when they were younger. If we live long enough, many of us (but certainly not all) will become truly cognitively impaired at some point and lose our ability to reason rationally, that wondrous quality that separates us from the other members of the animal kingdom.

The physiological or psychological conditions that can lead to cognitive impairment include not only reversible causes of memory loss, but also stroke, Alzheimer's disease, Parkinson's disease, certain types of tumors, cardiovascular problems, schizophrenia, and severe anxiety. These and many other disorders may produce symptoms of cognitive impairment. Your doctor should be able to determine whether your cognitive changes result from a reversible condition and help you to treat them effectively if they do.

However, certain other conditions affecting mental processes are harder to reverse. For example, mild neurocognitive disorder can often be the harbinger of other changes to come. It is present when you are experiencing small but noticeable alterations in your ability to think. People with it can continue to function relatively normally, but this condition isn't necessarily benign, as it progresses to some form of dementia within five years in about

50 percent of people with these cognitive changes. To see if you have any signs of it, have someone test you using the Saint Louis University Mental Status (SLUMS) Examination that Dr. John helped to develop, given in the appendix. If you want to know your chances of progression, have a brain MRI done to determine the volume of your hippocampus, the part of the brain that regulates memory, as small hippocampal volumes are predictive of future declines.

Moreover, approximately half of us will, if we live long enough, also develop some level of dementia. By definition, dementia means memory loss plus deficits in one or more areas of cognition. To be diagnosed with dementia, you must be unable to carry out some of your normal functioning, such as no longer being able to handle your finances, to work, or to take medications properly. While our loss of thought processes is not likely to greatly worry us personally (due to our lesser ability to think), it will certainly be traumatic for our friends and relatives.

The most devastating form of dementia is called Lewy body dementia and occurs in about one in ten cases. Its impact is potentially the most damaging because the people it afflicts have behavior problems early in the disease process. In one case, a deacon with Lewy body dementia, who had been happily married for forty years, started to make sexually inappropriate remarks to members of his congregation and undress in public! Unexplained angry outbursts by individuals with this type of dementia can also increase well in advance of memory decline.

Dementia itself has many potential causes, such as high blood pressure resulting in vascular changes that reduce blood flow to the brain (common in diabetes). The most usual cause of dementia, however, is Alzheimer's disease, making Alzheimer's just one of the different types of dementias, although the onset and progression vary with the origin. Alzheimer's disease is not as common as people believe. Only one in a hundred people in their sixties develops this disease; in people in their seventies, the incidence is only two or three per hundred. The numbers are only significantly higher when people reach their eighties and nineties.

Unfortunately, the drugs available to treat dementia work poorly, so little can be done to reverse its symptoms, aside from treating the reversible causes of memory loss in case any of them are contributing to the severity of the dementia. For individuals with diabetes, reducing the severity of vascular problems can provide greater blood flow to the brain and potentially improve their symptoms.

Action Steps for Better Health Tip #31

Mild neurocognitive disorder involves small alterations in your ability to think and may progress to dementia, characterized by memory loss plus deficits in one or more areas of cognition. Drugs to treat dementia work poorly, so the best approach is to simply treat the reversible causes of memory loss.

New Insights into Alzheimer's Disease

Alzheimer's disease is a disease that many fear getting, but relatively few will. If you have dealt with an aging relative with Alzheimer's, you have firsthand experience of how bad it can be. It essentially causes family members to mourn twice: first when they lose mental contact with the person they know and love, and again when that person dies much later. Undeniably, it's a devastating disorder of the brain that leads to memory loss, alterations in behavior and personality, inability to think appropriately, and loss of function.

This disease was first described by the pathologist, Alois Alzheimer, at the beginning of the twentieth century. He associated the changes in memory with the presence of amyloid plaques and neurofibrillary tangles in the brain (more on these later). While the majority of people who develop Alzheimer's disease are older, it can occur in middle age. Some individuals die in the first few years after diagnosis, but most survive eight to ten years and a few as long as twenty. At present, about four million Americans have it. Over the last decade, researchers have markedly enhanced knowledge about Alzheimer's disease. We can only look forward to seeing further breakthroughs in the near future that will lead to an enhanced quality of life for anyone developing this debilitating disease.

What Causes Alzheimer's Disease?

At present, there are two major theories about the cause of Alzheimer's disease. First, overproduction of beta-amyloid, a brain molecule produced in nerve cells, directly inhibits the ability to learn and recall events and also sets in motion a cascade of events that leads to brain tissue destruction. Dr. John and other researchers have found that in some cases beta-amyloid accumulates excessively in the human brain, leading to a buildup of toxic products and memory loss. The second theory is that this disease occurs when oxygen free radicals cause nerve degeneration. As evidence of this process, treatment with a free radical scavenger, alpha-lipoic acid (discussed in Step 1), leads to improved memory. But supplementing with vitamin E, a less potent antioxidant, has yielded mixed results. Research suggests that the two potential causes are likely linked.

Likewise, systemic inflammation may contribute to the onset of Alzheimer's disease. Elevated levels of ineffective insulin, found in an insulin-resistant state, are more common in people with vascular disease and type 2 diabetes. Even if you don't have diabetes, having elevated insulin levels increases your risk of Alzheimer's disease and memory deficits. Thus, Alzheimer's disease may actually prove to be another form of diabetes ("type 3"), because brain cells make some of their own insulin, but this hormone disappears early and dramatically in people with this disease, the result being a decreased clearance of beta-amyloid. It's unclear if lack of insulin or decreased insulin action in the brain occurs only locally or results from a lower insulin action in the rest of the body, but it is well established that poorly controlled diabetes increases your risk of mental decline and Alzheimer's. There is hope: you likely can improve your mental status by achieving control over your diabetes using medications such as insulin sensitizers.

The health of your cardiovascular system is also very important to the vitality of your brain. Your risk of developing Alzheimer's disease increases with the number of vascular risk factors that you have, such as insulin resistance, diabetes, smoking, hypertension, and heart disease. Diabetes by itself confers a greatly exaggerated risk of vascular complications and mental decline.

Is It Possible to Slow, Reverse, or Prevent Alzheimer's Disease?

Right now, ongoing research attempting to slow the overproduction of beta-amyloid offers great hope for more effective treatment and prevention of Alzheimer's disease in the near future. A number of potentially reversible factors may accelerate the onset of Alzheimer's, including a low education level, less diverse and intense recreational activities, lower physical activity, high levels of homocysteine (related to inadequate intake of vitamins B_6, B_{12}, and folate), and an underactive thyroid gland. An Australian study even concluded that people who pick their noses regularly are more likely to develop Alzheimer's disease.

At present, the safest way to prevent the onset of this disease is to participate in regular physical activity to slow your rate of brain tissue loss. Exercise also helps control blood glucose levels in people with diabetes and lower insulin levels in the blood by reversing insulin resistance. In addition, mental activity also delays potential declines in cognitive function, so make sure to regularly practice the mental exercises given earlier in this step.

Action Steps for Better Health Tip #32

Alzheimer's disease is one form of dementia but not the only potential cause. The onset of Alzheimer's is sometimes preventable. The best strategies to prevent its onset include regular physical activity and mental exercises, along with better control of your cardiovascular risk factors, such as insulin resistance, diabetes, and high blood pressure.

Drugs to Treat and Slow the Progression of Alzheimer's

To date, the treatment options for this disease leave a lot to be desired. One of the major neurotransmitters (i.e., substances that conduct nerve impulses) involved in the memory deficits seen in Alzheimer's disease is acetylcholine (ACh). Some of the available drugs, such as Aricept, block its breakdown, although none currently works very well. Other therapies have been investigated, but have also proven to be unsuccessful, including estrogen replacement and the use of nonsteroidal anti-inflammatory drugs like naproxen.

Are there any alternate therapies for this disease? As discussed in Step 3, testosterone levels slowly decline over one's lifetime. A number of studies, including Dr. John's, have found that this occurrence is associated with a lessening mental function, that visual-spatial memory can be enhanced with testosterone replacement, and that low testosterone levels are associated with Alzheimer's disease. In mice, testosterone reduces the production of amyloid precursor protein. In addition, ginkgo biloba is a medicinal herbal substance that appears to have some memory-enhancing effects in animals as well, but it hasn't been rigorously studied in humans yet. Finally, nootropics, or so-called smart drugs that improve blood flow in the brain, are inexpensive and appear to be about as effective in improving mental function as are the modern drugs.

Ghrelin, Hunger, and Mental Health

Ghrelin, the hormone produced in the stomach that signals when you're hungry (discussed in Step 3), may not make your body release more growth hormone, but it naturally helps you remember and learn things. This recent discovery could point to a new direction for a treatment for Alzheimer's disease: ghrelin replacement therapy to restore memory. Not surprising to most of us, there appears to be a direct link between the stomach and the brain. The latest research by Dr. John and others at Saint Louis University shows that high levels of ghrelin, the primary hormone that regulates appetite, trigger activity in the part of the brain responsible for learning and memory performance. In these studies, mice that lacked the ghrelin gene failed to do as well on behavioral tests, but when they received ghrelin replacement therapy, their memory improved and their ability to learn was restored. Thus ghrelin likely has a physiological role in maintaining memory. In fact, the ghrelin response could date back to the time when man had to forage for food when hungry. If you can't remember where your dinner ran off to, you'll have nothing to eat, so a better memory is ultimately important to the long-term survival of our species.

The Importance of Spirituality and Religion in Aging Well

We are just now beginning to fully recognize the role of spirituality and religion in the preservation of psychological and physical health throughout our lifetimes. Overall, both improve psychological health with a lesser effect on physical aspects of health, although not all forms of religion have positive effects. Their main role in health likely is to increase coping skills and enhance access to external support. For example, prayer is a commonly used coping strategy for anyone dealing with disability or life-threatening illnesses. People of all ages also seek to find meaning in their lives. Expressing spirituality through religious practice, compassion, service to others, or passing on wisdom to succeeding generations may bring deep personal satisfaction, comfort, and a sense of peace. Similarly, religious individuals generally live longer and function better, although people don't necessarily become more religious as they get older.

Action Steps for Better Health Tip #33

Both spirituality and religion can help you live the rest of your life with a greater sense of well-being. You don't have to be religious to experience spirituality, but both can help you deal more positively with adversity (e.g., changes in your body over time or illness) and give a deeper meaning to your life.

What We Know About Religion

Many people think that spirituality and religion are one and the same. You may experience both, but even though everyone has a spiritual component, not everyone is religious. One definition of religion is "a set of beliefs, values and practices based on the teachings of a spiritual leader." As defined, it would suggest that religion is a subset of a larger rubric called spirituality and religion is generally an organized expression of spirituality. Religion offers a way to express spirituality with social support, security, and a sense of belonging through religious affiliations, all of which are important to coping with adversity. Religion is also steeped with tradition, which becomes more important to people the longer they live.

What We Know About Spirituality

Although religion may include specific beliefs and practices, spirituality is far broader. Defining spirituality, therefore, is a bit like describing color to a blind person who has never known sight. Your perception of your spiritual self will vary according to your beliefs. Spirituality is more about being concerned with things of the spirit—the big questions of meaning, metaphysics, and existence. Being spiritual is thinking about, wondering about, and exploring the deepest aspects of reality, values, morals, and meanings, but it should never be equated with supernaturalism. It's about all the ways that we try to make sense of living and our attempts to make good come from our lives and actions. Spiritual development provides us with insight and understanding of ourselves and others.

Strategies to Bring Spirituality into Your Life

Spiritual awakening is a journey, and you may feel the call to embark on a spiritual path after going through a difficult time or when certain parts of your life are no longer flowing as smoothly as they once did. Sharing your unique, personal experiences, even if they are outside of traditional realms, can increase your feelings of spirituality. Talking about your dreams, daydreams, near-death experiences, visions, hallucinations, and more serves as a positive outlet for your emotions.

Similarly, feelings of hope are associated with a longer life. Hope may be used as a means of coping with changes occurring to your body over time because it can improve your expectations for the future, motivate you to take action, or give you the means of fulfilling your goals. Religious and spiritual activity can even help you recover faster from illness or injury.

Finally, creating legacies is another very constructive approach to bringing meaning and spirituality into your life. They may be expressed as written or recorded memoirs, photograph collections, memory gardens, family histories or genealogies, and autobiographies or life histories. For some, making trips to family homes or pilgrimages to locations of spiritual significance also increase positive feelings. For others, telephone calls, prayer circles, televised religious services, and sacred readings may offer hope and solace.

As far as your physical health is concerned, making the effort to attend church services regularly is far better than simply watching televangelists without leaving your home. People who go to churches, mosques, or synagogues tend to maintain their physical and mental function longer than those who don't. Just getting out of the house and getting some exercise may explain some of these differences.

A Definitive Study on Positive Mental Health Factors

Professor George Valiant at Harvard University followed a group of Harvard graduates from age fifty to eighty years and a group of inner-city dwellers from age fifty to seventy. He found that a number of mental health factors not only were strongly related to survival, but also distinguished who became the "happy-well" as opposed to the "sad-sick" as they aged. Positive mental factors were the ability to deal with adversity, being in a stable marriage, getting some exercise, not smoking, not abusing alcohol, and not becoming overweight. Exercise, especially resistance exercise, decreased depression. Perhaps we can all learn something from this study about how to become one of the happy-well people throughout the rest of our long lives.

A Final Word About Step 4

Not every memory lapse signals bigger problems, and certainly not everyone is going to end up with dementia or Alzheimer's disease. Treat depression, check out spirituality, and continue being creative for best lifelong results. Our additional suggestions for allowing your mind to stay young for longer are to manage your crises well, enjoy a stable marriage, exercise regularly, avoid smoking, use alcohol only moderately, watch your weight—and do some crossword puzzles or other equally mentally challenging activities. Have your kids or grandkids teach you how to do the new craze of "number crosswords" called Sudoku or some of their fast-paced video games—your mind will love you for it!

Maintain a Stable Weight

"Everything I eat has been proved by some data or other to be a deadly poison, and everything I don't eat has been proved to be indispensable to life. But I go marching on."

—*George Bernard Shaw (1856–1950)*

Too fat, too thin, just right—how do you know where your body weight falls? We are continually bombarded with messages about how fat Americans have become and how bad this weight gain is for our nation's health. Interestingly, while the United States became the fattest nation in the world during the twentieth century, our average life span still increased by twenty-seven years. This conundrum makes us realize that nothing is ever quite what it appears or is as simple as we would like it to be. In some cases, weight loss can be good (if it's fat weight alone), but it can also be bad if what you're losing is your muscle mass instead. In fact, sarcopenia, the medical term for muscle wasting, can vastly decrease your quality of life and make you feel older than you actually are.

This important step lets you know how to tell if your body weight is appropriate. It additionally gives practical suggestions to help you maintain a healthy and stable weight, primarily through increased physical activity and early medical interventions, the goal of which is to make you look and feel as good as possible at any age.

Good and Bad News About Your Weight

The good news is that as you get older, being *slightly* overweight may actually improve how long and well you live. However, we're certainly not advising you to allow yourself to sit around and gain weight, since the bad news is that for adults in their middle years, expanding waistlines are associated with type 2 diabetes, hypertension, and heart disease. Excess body fat has become the "wicked witch" of modern medicine. We contend, however, that body fat has gotten a bad rap that it likely does not fully deserve. In fact, after sixty years of age, significant weight loss is actually bad for most people and usually not recommended.

Body fat is a powerfully active metabolic tissue in the body that produces a variety of hormones, such as leptin and adiponectin, as well as cytokines that can be both good and bad (more on these later). Although excess fat is often directly blamed for type 2 diabetes onset, a *minor* loss of weight (only 5 to 7 percent of your total weight, equivalent to about ten or so pounds for a two-hundred-pound person) can vastly improve blood glucose levels and overall diabetes control, as long as what you lose is body fat and not muscle. What's more, people without much subcutaneous fat (located right below the skin's surface) often develop a condition known as lipoatrophic diabetes, a type of diabetes caused by having too little fat.

In addition to having important metabolic activity, fat plays an important role in protecting your vital organs. Likewise, a fatty cushion around your hips helps protect them from being fractured if you fall. It also acts as insulation, keeping you warm in colder environments. Perhaps most important, fat acts as a storage organ, just as the camel's hump allows it to travel long distances without eating or drinking, which can be vitally important if you suffer through a prolonged illness or long stay in the hospital at any point in your life.

It's unlikely that body fat is the direct or sole cause of all the health conditions for which it gets blamed, although it appears to contribute to a certain degree. Whether you lose weight or not, fat cells become more responsive to insulin after endurance training, as do muscle cells. Both types of cells are thought to contribute heavily to insulin resistance and the development of type 2 diabetes. Moreover, a recent study concluded that obesity per se is not a direct risk factor for organ failure or premature death, but having diabetes can be.

Action Steps for Better Health Tip #34

Having too little body fat can often be as bad for you as having too much. For a number of reasons, major weight loss is not advised after you reach the age of sixty. So if you're not there yet, now is the time to prevent getting too much abdominal (central) fat that can harm your health, by exercising more and changing your diet for the better. If you are trying to lose weight, make certain to exercise regularly to retain your muscle mass.

Too Much Weight Loss Can Be Bad for You

One main problem with large amounts of weight loss after you reach middle age or older is that these losses consist of about 75 percent fat and 25 percent muscle for typical dieters, but when you gain weight back afterward (which is extremely common within six months to a year), a larger percentage (up to 85 percent) of your lost weight is regained as body fat. Having less muscle also lowers your caloric needs, making it easier to gain weight even when you're eating the same number of calories after your diet as you were consuming beforehand. Furthermore, people who yo-yo diet over their lifetimes (frequently cycling between weight loss and regain) eventually will have insufficient muscle left to carry their extra weight, making them become one of the "fat frail" likely to have a reduced quality of life resulting from their inadequate strength.

Therefore, if you are losing any body weight, it's essential that you regularly exercise to maintain your muscle mass. In fact, when it comes to maintaining a good body weight and your health, physical activity is likely more important than how many calories you eat. Dieters who fail to exercise lose more muscle mass, but exercise during periods of restricted calorie intake stimulates the retention of your muscle, which also keeps your metabolism operating at a higher level.

Another significant problem is that when you diet and try to lose excessive amounts of body weight, you can easily develop a condition know as protein energy malnutrition, which results from inadequate intake of calories, especially from protein sources. When present, it can lead to physical problems (e.g., pressure ulcers, anemia, hip fractures, infections, and muscle weakness) that can make your health suffer. It compromises your immune function, which is already negatively impacted somewhat by your getting older. For example, this type of malnutrition can lead to a marked decrease in your CD4 T cells, which are important disease-fighting immune cells. In fact, CD4 T cell levels can become as low as those seen in AIDS patients, opening up the door for unusual infections and a greater potential need for extended use of antibiotic treatments.

Weight loss causes triglycerides, which are stored fats, to come out of your body fat and liver cells. Released into the blood, these fats can add to the bad type of cholesterol, potentially contributing to heart disease, arterial plaque formation, and blood clots. Another consideration is that when losing excess fat, you also release whatever has been stored in your fat tissue, including a lifetime of accumulated toxins like PCBs and DDEs from insecticides. This rapid increase in levels of circulating toxins can actually lead to nerve damage. In the natural world, bald eagles rapidly die when they lose weight, due to the toxins in their brains that get released. This "poisonous infusion" may be the major reason why weight loss at an older age (when you have had a longer time for toxins to accumulate) is bad for you. Along the same lines, many medications are also stored in fat tissue, and weight loss releases more of them into your bloodstream. Most physicians fail to reduce the dosage of fat-soluble drugs during periods of weight loss, likely making the doses that you're exposed to excessively high.

In some people, excessive weight loss is just a harbinger of diseases such as cancer, particularly when the weight loss is unintended and unexpected. If you find yourself losing a lot of weight without trying to, you should see your doctor to rule out disease as a potential cause—while it's still early enough to treat. Even if you're trying to lose some weight, it likely may not be in your best interest to do so once you're older than sixty: even intentional weight loss in older women results in more than twice the risk of hip fractures, frailty, and nursing home admissions. As you can see, there are many good reasons not to attempt to lose significant amounts of weight once you get past a certain age.

What Is a Healthy Weight?

The influence of weight on longevity and optimal health has been well studied, and it appears that a modest weight gain throughout life may be healthy. A gain of about ten pounds per decade, depending upon the size of your skeleton and the amount of muscle you have, is usually permissable, but the actual acceptable amount will vary from person to person.

Using Body Mass Index as Your Guide

The currently favored method for body weight assessment is the body mass index (BMI), which is used to determine ideal body weight (see Table 5.1, on the next page). BMI, like body weight, follows a U-shaped curve; that is, both very low and very high BMI values appear to be more risky as far as your long-term health is concerned, so it's not good to be too thin or excessively overweight. However, there is a slight rise in the healthiest BMI range as people get older, from an average BMI of 21.4 for twenty- to twenty-nine-year-olds up to 26.6 for sixty- to sixty-nine-year-olds, which is not

TABLE 5.1 Body Mass Index and Healthy Weights for Adults

BODY WEIGHT (POUNDS)

BMI	Healthy Weight						Overweight						Obese				
	19	20	21	22	23	24	25	26	27	28	29	30	31	32	33	34	35
4'10"	91	96	100	105	110	115	119	124	129	134	138	143	148	153	158	162	167
4'11"	94	99	104	109	114	119	124	128	133	138	143	148	153	158	163	168	173
5'0"	97	102	107	112	118	123	128	133	138	143	148	153	158	163	168	174	179
5'1"	100	106	111	116	122	127	132	137	143	148	153	158	164	169	174	180	185
5'2"	104	109	115	120	126	131	136	142	147	153	158	164	169	175	180	186	191
5'3"	107	113	118	124	130	135	141	146	152	158	163	169	175	180	186	191	197
5'4"	110	116	122	128	134	140	145	151	157	163	169	174	180	186	192	197	204
5'5"	114	120	126	132	138	144	150	156	162	168	174	180	186	192	198	204	210
5'6"	118	124	130	136	142	148	155	161	167	173	179	186	192	198	204	210	216
5'7"	121	127	134	140	146	153	159	166	172	178	185	191	198	204	211	217	223
5'8"	125	131	138	144	151	158	164	171	177	184	190	197	203	210	216	223	230
5'9"	128	135	142	149	155	162	169	176	182	189	196	203	209	216	223	230	236
5'10"	132	139	146	153	160	167	174	181	188	195	202	209	216	222	229	236	243
5'11"	136	143	150	157	165	172	179	186	193	200	208	215	222	229	236	243	250
6'0"	140	147	154	162	169	177	184	191	199	206	213	221	228	235	242	250	258
6'1"	144	151	159	166	174	182	189	197	204	212	219	227	235	242	250	257	265
6'2"	148	155	163	171	179	186	194	202	210	218	225	233	241	249	256	264	272
6'3"	152	160	168	176	184	192	200	208	216	224	232	240	248	256	264	272	279
6'4"	156	164	172	180	189	197	205	213	221	230	238	246	254	263	271	279	287

HEIGHT

reflected in the values in the table. The BMI values in Table 5.1 are really most appropriate for people in younger age ranges, but ranges for older individuals have not yet been published.

Another drawback of using this method, aside from the age issue, is that if you are rather muscular, your BMI may not reflect the added healthiness that muscle bestows, as your BMI value reveals nothing about your actual body composition (body fat versus muscle). Muscle mass weighs more than fat for the same volume, so having extra muscle mass will raise your BMI. An added problem with using BMI is that experts now contend that healthy ranges may vary by ethnic groups and are usually higher for African Americans and lower for Asians. The table is usually accurate for Caucasians, though, in particular the younger ones.

Calculating Your BMI

You can easily calculate your BMI. It equals your weight in kilograms divided by the square of your height in meters (wt/ht^2). Take your weight in pounds and divide by 2.2 to get your weight in kilograms, along with your height in inches multiplied by 0.0254 to get your height in meters. For example, if you weigh 75 kg (165 pounds) and you are 1.75 meters tall (5 feet, 9 inches), your BMI is the following: $75/1.75^2 = 75/3.06 = 24.5$. Alternatively, you can use pounds and inches in the equation and simply multiply the answer by 705. You can also find BMI calculators online, such as the one provided by the National Institutes of Health at nhlbisupport.com/bmi/bmicalc.htm.

Where You Store Your Excess Body Fat Matters

With regard to staying healthy, it matters not only how much excess body fat you have, but also where you store it. Obesity comes in two types: abdominal (central) and peripheral (lower body), also known as android and gynoid obesity, respectively. In central obesity, the excess fat tissue is concentrated in the abdominal, neck, shoulder, and arm areas, making a person apple-shaped, which is more typical in males. Much of this fat is stored within the abdomen, in and around your organs. On the other hand, gynoid obesity is more common in females and involves carrying extra weight in the hips, thighs, and buttocks, causing a person to be pear-shaped. Of the two, central obesity is far more dangerous to your health. Body fat storage, unfortunately, is genetically predetermined, and you control only the total amount of fat that you store, not where you put it.

Action Steps for Better Health Tip #35

Where you store your excess body fat can impact your health. Carrying extra fat weight in your abdominal region has potentially dire health consequences. You control only how much fat you store, not where it goes, so prevention of excessive weight gain is the most effective strategy for achieving and maintaining optimal health and youthful vigor.

Using a Tape Measure May Prolong Your Life

In addition to measuring your weight and (BMI), you should also follow your waist-to-hip ratio (WHR), as it will give you feedback about whether you're storing too much abdominal fat to maintain good health. Due to inherent anatomical differences between men and women, optimal WHR differs by sex. A high WHR in either sex is the result of central obesity. This more metabolically active "visceral fat" is easier to gain and lose, but it's also commonly associated with metabolic disorders such as insulin resistance, type 2 diabetes, high blood pressure, heart disease, and more. In fact, a higher WHR may ultimately affect brain structures and speed your development of cognitive declines and dementia.

Obesity is most risky for men whose WHR is greater than 1 and for women whose WHR is greater than 0.85. A WHR of less than or equal to 0.9 reduces metabolic risk for most men, while 0.8 is the cutoff for women. In people of Chinese origin, the ideal cutoff for men is lower, between 0.8 and 0.85. Just waist circumference alone may be predictive of type 2 diabetes risk. Men with waists that are 37.9 to 39.8 inches in circumference, for example, have a fivefold greater risk of developing diabetes than men whose waists are 29 to 34 inches, likely due to increased visceral fat storage. Women's waists should be less than 34.7 inches to lower their diabetes risk.

You May Be Fatter than You Think

At present, only a minority of the American population meets recommended weight categories, so if you're comparing yourself with everyone around you, you may think your body size is normal. Nearly a third of adults are obese, and more than two-thirds are overweight, which also means that many already will be overly fat when reaching the age of sixty. As a nation, some of the feedback that let us know when we were gaining weight has been taken away. Nowadays, pants are made with adjustable waist fittings, and jeans are made with stretchy material, which expands to fit when we eat too much. Furthermore, clothing manufacturers recently made a woman's dress size 10 today that is the equivalent of size 14 from a few decades ago (without telling anyone). So you can't tell anymore if you're gaining too much fat weight by whether you still fit in the same size of women's clothing. If you're going to

Measuring Your Waist-to-Hip Ratio Accurately

To measure your WHR accurately, you need to take your measurements (in inches or centimeters) at specific sites. Your waist is measured as the circumference at your belly button, while hip measures are taken around the widest part of your buttocks. Watching the change in your measurements over time will provide better information than just watching your weight. A reduction in your waist measurement will likely enhance your life expectancy and improve your health.

use how your clothes fit as your gauge, pick one pair of pants that you already own (ignoring the size label) to assess changes in your girth over time.

Losing Weight Is Only Half the Battle

If you haven't reached your sixtieth birthday yet, now is the time to think about increasing your exercise and modifying your diet to lose as much of your abdominal fat as you possibly can. To do so, any diet will work as long as you eat fewer calories than your body needs. The most important thing is to lose fat instead of muscle by including exercise in your daily routine while you're dieting. Your actual scale weight losses may be slower with the exercise added in (since you're gaining muscle), but your body composition will be changing for the better. Also, avoid diets with really low calorie intakes that cause rapid or extreme weight loss. They result in greater losses of body water and muscle, which adds to the ease of regaining weight once you're back to eating normally.

Keeping yourself from regaining lost weight is usually a bigger challenge than losing it in the first place. Even among successful dieters, over 90 percent regain the same amount (or more) within six months to a year. How can you keep the weight off? You will need to make permanent lifestyle changes that will benefit both your weight and your health. A lot can be learned from the National Weight Control Registry, which for over a decade has tracked people who lost at least thirty pounds and kept it off for at least a year. Their results confirm what exercise physiologists, like Dr. Sheri, have known all along: physical activity is critical for weight maintenance, particularly after weight loss. Almost all of the successful participants have continued using up about 2,000 calories a week doing a regular physical activity like walking (i.e., 60 minutes of brisk walking five to six days a week on average) to keep their weight down. Other lifestyle habits are important as well, such as being conscientious about what you eat (i.e., more healthful food in appropriate portions) and starting the day off right with a healthy breakfast. Interestingly, regularly eating breakfast also lowers your risk of developing diabetes.

Action Steps for Better Health Tip #36

The keys to losing the type of weight you want to lose—fat, not muscle—and keeping it off are doing daily exercise, even if it's just brisk walking; continuing to watch what you eat; and starting your day by eating a healthy breakfast.

Why Loss of Appetite and Weight Are More Common the Older You Get

As we've discussed, excessive weight loss is a serious concern once you're past sixty because it is associated with a lower quality of life and more frequent health problems like hip fractures. It can occur for many reasons as you age, but a key factor is your diminishing appetite. In ancient Roman times, Cicero pointed out, "I am grateful to old age because it has increased my desire for good conversation and decreased my interest in good food." However, losing your appetite when you're getting older usually is not a good thing to have happen.

The concept of a physiological anorexia associated with advancing age, as first hypothesized by Dr. John in 1988, is now well established. After you reach a certain age (which differs for everyone but can include the forties), you likely will find that your appetite is not as robust as it was when you were younger, and your sense of taste and smell may be blunted, which can lower your enjoyment of foods. The keys to reversing excessive weight loss due to lack of appetite are eating multiple small meals to overcome a sense of stomach fullness and taking caloric supplements between meals.

It's important that you maintain your caloric intake because appetite problems, if untreated, can lead to muscle wasting. If your goal is to live a long time while feeling as youthful as you can, you should at all costs avoid letting your muscles waste away.

Thankfully, many causes of appetite loss are reversible. Taking multiple medications can reduce your appetite, but you also can talk with your doctor about trying other medications, lowering dosages, or taking ones with less of an appetite-suppressive effect. Likewise, chronic pain and multiple illnesses can make eating less appealing or more difficult, but all of these issues can be controlled or fixed through medical means. Feeling depressed also can cause appetite loss at any age and should be treated sooner than later if for no other reason than that. Other reversible causes of appetite loss include alcoholism, swallowing problems, and low-salt or low-cholesterol diets, which have less flavor. If your desire to eat isn't fixed by reversing these problems, appetite-enhancing drugs are available to try, such as Megace ES (megestrol acetate), which has the side benefit of decreasing cytokine production while enhancing appetite and weight gain.

Action Steps for Better Health Tip #37

Weight loss can easily occur if your appetite becomes less robust than it used to be. Prevent excessive weight loss by eating adequate calories and protein in small meals and by exercising regularly, including doing some resistance training. Also, treating reversible causes of appetite or weight loss can usually correct the problem.

A Pivotal Role for Cytokines in Weight Loss and Sarcopenia

Cytokines are peptides (small proteins) produced by all body cells for their own protection and include interleukins, interferons, tumor necrosis factors, transforming growth factor-beta, and cellular stimulating factors. The concept that the immune system produces substances that help cells communicate with one another was established long ago and is certainly not groundbreaking, but the recent discovery that cytokines have direct, positive effects on the healthiness of the central nervous system, muscle, bone, and other tissues is exciting. The more we learn about how they work, the more likely it is that we can use them to find a way to enhance long-term health.

On the flip side, an excess of cytokines can act as an inflammatory agent and cause illnesses, so you wouldn't want to start popping them even if they were available in pill form (luckily, they're not). Not only do they produce anorexia and sickness behavior when released in excess, but they also pull protein out of muscles and calcium out of bone, decrease red blood cells, interfere with memory, inhibit albumin production (a protein found in the bloodstream), and more. Classically, two of these compounds, interleukin-6 (IL-6) and tumor necrosis factor-alpha (TNF-alpha), tend to accelerate the physiological aging process and lead to a loss of muscle fibers.

Elevated levels of IL-6 increase your risk of experiencing a lower quality of living, particularly if you have rheumatoid arthritis, lung problems, or heart failure, because too much IL-6 causes reduced muscle mass and lost strength. Excess cytokines likely play a key role in sarcopenia, the muscle-wasting syndrome associated with a loss of strength, and in a greater incidence of health problems that limit your ability to continue feeling good your entire lifetime.

Action Steps for Better Health Tip #38

Elevated levels of compounds called cytokines can damage your muscles. While you can't completely prevent loss of muscle mass, you can combat muscle loss with resistance training, creatine supplements, testosterone, adequate amounts of calories and protein in your diet, and appetite-enhancing drugs.

Keep Your Muscles Strong

Although maintaining or even gaining muscle mass through training and supplementation can't completely prevent and reverse declines in your muscle strength over time, keeping what muscle mass you have and trying to gain more should remain your goal for looking and feeling younger for longer. At present, resistance exercise is the best treatment for restoring lost muscle mass, and doing such training at any age is also an excellent way to prevent muscle loss in the first place. Likewise, both creatine monohydrate and testosterone supplementation (discussed in Step 3) have shown some promise in reversing muscle wasting. Normally, your muscles are in a constant state of flux with muscle hypertrophy (increase in mass) balancing out muscle atrophy (loss). Anabolic hormones such as testosterone appear to produce beneficial effects by stimulating hypertrophy while inhibiting atrophy. Testosterone can also stimulate muscle repair, but remember that atrophy is driven largely by elevated cytokine levels, along with protein malnutrition, so making sure you eat adequate amounts of calories and protein will help as well.

Identify the Potential for Weight Loss Early

By the time you've reached the age of sixty, it's dangerous to use the watch-and-wait approach if you start losing weight. However, losing a lot of muscle mass when you're younger than sixty can also result in a loss of vitality and good health. To assess your risk sooner rather than later, Dr. John and others have created a four-question screening tool that can indicate whether a poor appetite is likely to cause excessive loss of weight and muscle. More than eight times out of ten, scores on the Simplified Nutritional Appetite Questionnaire (SNAQ, pronounced "snack") can identify who will go on to lose 5 percent or more of body weight. The test is even more sensitive in predicting who will lose 10 percent, as it identifies the problem 88 percent of the time, and it is equally reliable for old and young. The questionnaire takes less than two minutes to complete.

SNAQ: The Simplified Nutritional Assessment Questionnaire

1. My appetite is
   a. very poor
   b. poor
   c. average
   d. good
   e. very good

2. When I eat,
   a. I feel full after eating only a few mouthfuls
   b. I feel full after eating about a third of a meal
   c. I feel full after eating over half a meal
   d. I feel full after eating most of the meal
   e. I hardly ever feel full

3. Food tastes
   a. very bad
   b. bad
   c. average
   d. good
   e. very good

4. Normally I eat
   a. less than one meal a day
   b. one meal a day
   c. two meals a day
   d. three meals a day
   e. more than three meals a day

Tally the SNAQ results based on the following numerical scale: a = 1, b = 2, c = 3, d = 4, e = 5. The sum of the scores for the individual items constitutes the SNAQ score. A SNAQ score of less than 14 indicates significant risk of at least 5 percent weight loss within six months and should prompt a trip to the doctor and a nutritional assessment.

A Final Word About Step 5

It's acceptable to be slightly overweight as you get older, just not excessively so. Being too fat is associated with health problems that can make you feel older sooner, but so is being too thin, particularly if you have experienced significant muscle losses. Regular exercise is the best strategy for fat weight loss, body weight maintenance, and retention of muscle mass. To prevent reversible loss of appetite and muscle mass, seek medical interventions if you find your appetite diminishing. Some of these problems can be resolved with prescription medications to enhance appetite or muscle. To date, the most effective treatment of muscle loss is resistance training to stimulate your body to gain and retain muscle mass fibers.

Love Your Healthy Heart

"We know a great deal more about the causes of physical disease than we do about the causes of physical health."

—*M. Scott Peck (1936–2005) in* The Road Less Traveled

How can you keep your heart in good working order? The four most common types of cardiovascular disease (CVD)—coronary heart disease (which includes heart attack and chest pain), stroke, high blood pressure, and heart failure—and their causes are discussed in detail in this step. By learning more about each, you will know how to lower your risk of ever developing them. For example, simply living a sedentary lifestyle is a strong risk factor for heart disease, and you can lower or remove this risk by becoming physically active.

Similarly, many blood fat abnormalities such as elevated cholesterol levels (another risk factor) can be managed through greater consumption of fish and dark chocolate, drinking moderate amounts of alcohol, and sensibly approaching the use of medications for cholesterol, blood pressure, and diabetes. In this step, you'll learn to love your healthy heart. By taking better care of it, you can enhance your longevity and increase your odds of living a long and healthy life with your heart and arteries throughout your body in good working order.

Which Cardiovascular Diseases Are Most Common?

Taken all together, cardiovascular events are the leading cause of death for Americans, accounting for about half annually. Individually, heart disease and stroke are the most common CVDs, ones that often lead to a lower quality of life, an older biological age, and a shortened life span. More than 70 million Americans currently live with some form of CVD.

Although these health conditions are more common among people older than sixty-five, the number of sudden deaths from heart disease among people between fifteen and thirty-four years old has recently increased with declines in health attributable to unhealthy lifestyle choices. The good news is that if lifestyle choices are causing an increased incidence of such problems, then these problems more than likely can be prevented or reversed by similar means: by improving diet and increasing physical activity.

What Is Coronary Heart Disease?

Heart disease is caused by atherosclerosis, which occurs when the inner walls of the coronary arteries become narrowed due to a buildup of plaque filled with fat, cholesterol, calcium and other substances. *Atherosclerosis* comes from the Greek words *athero*, meaning "gruel" or "paste," and *sclerosis*, meaning "hardness." When this process causes a partial or complete blockage of the arteries feeding the heart (the coronary arteries), it results in what is known as coronary artery or coronary heart disease.

Plaque formations can grow large enough to significantly reduce the ability of the blood to flow through an artery, but most heart damage occurs when plaque becomes fragile and ruptures, causing blood clots to form. A clot that blocks a blood vessel feeding the heart causes a heart attack. Such clots often occur in coronary vessels that are less than 50 percent blocked, which means heart attacks can happen even if your plaque accumulation is not significant. If a clot blocks blood flow for long enough, the part of the heart muscle that is not receiving enough blood through the blocked artery ends up infarcting, or dying.

If blockage is detected early enough, physicians may use balloon angioplasty to force arteries open or implantable steel screens called stents, which are mechanical devices to hold open clogged vessels, in an attempt to restore more normal blood flow through affected coronary arteries. Many individuals with diagnosed heart disease are put on cholesterol-lowering drug therapies and may also be advised to make dietary and exercise lifestyle improvements.

Action Steps for Better Health Tip #39

You can lower your risk for developing heart disease by preventing, reversing, or controlling the main causes that are modifiable. These risk factors include cigarette smoking, elevated blood levels of bad cholesterol and triglycerides, high blood pressure, diabetes, obesity, and physical inactivity.

Major risk factors for heart disease include both modifiable ones that you can potentially improve and others that you can't change. For example, advancing age is a nonmodifiable risk factor, while diabetes is modifiable by improving your blood glucose control. Similarly, the risk of developing problems caused by cigarette smoking is greatly reduced by quitting cigarette consumption. Other modifications you can make to limit or lower your risk are discussed later in this step.

How Peripheral Artery Disease Can Affect the Legs

Peripheral artery disease (PAD) is a common circulatory problem that limits blood flow to the legs and arms. Plaque can form in any artery around the body, not just in the ones feeding the heart and the brain, and PAD usually occurs in peripheral arteries in the legs. Pain in the lower legs during walking is a common symptom, but you should also be aware that PAD can be a sign of widespread plaque formation in other arteries around the body. If plaque formations in leg arteries rupture, a blockage can occur, limiting or cutting off blood supply to the lower legs, and resulting in pain, changes in skin color, sores or ulcers, difficulty walking, and even gangrene.

PAD can be diagnosed by measuring your leg blood pressure and comparing it to measurements made on your arm. If they're unequal, you may have blockage in your lower limbs raising the pressure there. You can get your PAD under control and maintain your normal activities. Walking or other daily exercise is a key to maintaining optimal circulation in your legs, along with a healthy diet and smoking cessation. In addition, certain medications can cause dilation of your leg arteries, and surgery can be done to improve blood flow to your legs by bypassing blockages.

What Do You Need to Know About Strokes?

Every forty-five seconds, someone in America has a stroke, and about every fourth one is fatal. As mentioned, a stroke results from cardiovascular disease in the arteries leading to and within the brain. The brain is an extremely complex organ that controls various body functions. When a blood vessel carrying oxygen and nutrients to the brain is either blocked by a clot or bursts, part of the brain doesn't get the blood and oxygen it needs, resulting in a stroke in the affected region.

Strokes can have different origins. Flow blockages from clots cause ischemic strokes (which account for about 83 percent of all cases), while ruptured blood vessels that leak blood (i.e., hemorrhage) into the brain cause a hemorrhagic stroke. This second type is usually caused by either an aneurysm (a ballooning out of a vessel) or a vessel malformation. A stroke's impact can vary; only the functions normally controlled by the affected part of the brain will be impaired. One that reduces blood flow to the back of your brain, for instance, is likely to negatively impact your vision.

Other areas of the brain control movement, speech, memory, and problem-solving ability.

Action Steps for Better Health Tip #40

Ischemic strokes are the most common type. If blood flow to an area of the brain is reduced for any reason, normal functions controlled by that area will be impaired. If you have any symptoms of stroke, get to a hospital as quickly as you can to receive tPA (a clot-busting drug for ischemic stroke) for the best possible outcome.

The most promising treatment for ischemic stroke is the FDA-approved clot-busting drug tPA (tissue plasminogen activator), which must be administered within a three-hour window from the onset of symptoms to work effectively. If you have stroke symptoms, get to a hospital quickly to get this drug in time. To prevent strokes in the first place, you should consider taking anti-platelet agents such as aspirin and Plavix (clopidogrel) or anticoagulants like Coumadin (warfarin) that lower the risk of blood clot formation. If you have stomach ulcers or already take other anti-inflammatory drugs such as Advil or Motrin (ibuprofen), you should take no more than a baby aspirin (75 mg) a day. For most other people, taking 325 milligrams of a coated aspirin (Ecotrin) is good for stroke prevention.

Is a Transient Ischemic Attack a Form of Stroke?

Transient ischemic attacks (TIAs) are minor or warning strokes that usually result in typical stroke symptoms. Normal blood flow to the brain is only reduced for a short time and tends to resolve by itself. Even though the symptoms disappear after a short time, TIAs are strong indicators of a possible major stroke in the future. You should heed the warning and take steps immediately to prevent an actual, more damaging stroke, including seeking medical care by starting on clot-preventing medications and controlling high blood pressure.

React Quickly to Warning Signs of Heart Attack or Stroke

The most common heart attack symptom is chest pain or discomfort, but women are somewhat more likely than men to experience other symptoms, including shortness of breath, nausea and vomiting, and back or jaw pain (see the sidebar "Heart Attack Warning Signs"). Even if you're busy, you should stop to determine the source of mild chest pain rather than potentially ending up with a more damaging heart attack. In other words, always take any chest pain or discomfort seriously. When your heart is not receiving enough blood, lactic acid begins to build up, leading to pain or discomfort; lack of oxygen to your heart (and often to the other parts of your body) can cause additional symptoms, which should be a sign to you that something is wrong. People with diabetes can often suffer from symptom-free heart attacks, so even a sudden onset of extreme fatigue is a symptom that needs to be checked out.

Heart Attack Warning Signs

- **Lasting or intermittent chest discomfort in the center of the chest:** It sometimes feels like bad indigestion, or it can feel like uncomfortable pressure, squeezing, fullness, or acute and stabbing pain.
- **Pain or discomfort radiating down one or both arms, back, neck, jaw, or stomach:** This symptom is due to "referred pain," which is actually originating in the heart due to lack of adequate amounts of oxygen.
- **Shortness of breath, particularly when unusual or unexpected:** It can occur along with chest discomfort or without it.
- **Other symptoms:** Sudden sweating, nausea and vomiting, lightheadedness, or undue, unexplained fatigue are also warning signs.

Heed these warning signs, and seek medical attention imme-diately for the best possible outcome. If detected early, blood clots can often be dissolved, resulting in less lasting damage to your heart or other areas of your body. Don't wait more than five min-utes after your symptoms start to call for help, and don't waste pre-cious minutes by having someone drive you to a hospital. Using emergency medical services (EMS) by dialing 9-1-1 is the fastest and most effective way to get lifesaving medical attention.

If you are with someone who loses consciousness and stops breathing, he or she is experiencing cardiac arrest. Activate EMS, preferably by having someone else call for you, and begin cardio-pulmonary resuscitation (CPR) until help arrives.

Action Steps for Better Health Tip #41

Know the usual warning symptoms of heart attack or stroke. Don't delay in seeking immediate medical attention, preferably through activating EMS by calling 9-1-1. Lifesaving treatment in the first few minutes is critical for surviving and thriving with a minimum of lasting problems after a major cardiac event.

For stroke, the key word to describe its symptoms is sudden. If someone experiences any or all of the symptoms listed in the sidebar

Stroke Warning Signs

- Sudden numbness or weakness, especially on one side of the body (affecting the legs, arms, face, or elsewhere)
- Sudden confusion
- Sudden trouble with normal speaking or understanding
- Sudden loss of vision in one or both eyes
- Sudden trouble with walking, loss of balance, or lack of physical coordination
- Sudden onset, severe headache and dizziness

"Stroke Warning Signs," such as sudden numbness down one side of the body or trouble speaking, immediately call 9-1-1 (or your local EMS number, if different) to summon an ambulance with advanced life support. Taking immediate action is critical because if given within three hours of the start of symptoms, the clot-busting drug tPA can improve the long-term outcomes for most individuals.

Why Is High Blood Pressure a Silent Killer?

Blood pressure is defined as the force of the blood pushing against the walls of your arteries, which is recorded as two numbers, such as 122 over 78 mm of mercury (122/78 mm Hg). The first number is the higher, systolic, pressure exerted during heartbeats, which is the contraction of the heart muscle that forces blood into arteries. The second represents the lower, diastolic, pressure that occurs when your heart is resting between beats. High blood pressure, or hypertension, describes a condition in which your blood travels through your vasculature at pressures consistently above normal, usually diagnosed at 140/90 mm Hg for adults less than seventy years of age.

In older individuals, elevations of the systolic blood pressure are very common, and most studies have shown that simply keeping it below 160 mm Hg when you're getting older decreases stroke risk. Actually, over time people with low blood pressure often have poorer health, making a systolic pressure between 140 and 150 ideal for most individuals reaching their seventies (and even higher in their eighties). Blood pressure should be a little more

---

Action Steps for Better Health Tip #42

High blood pressure is a silent killer that you can control before it's too late. Lower your blood pressure readings by engaging in regular exercise, cutting back on salt, and taking prescribed medications to keep your systolic values less than 160 mm Hg.

tightly controlled in people with diabetes of any age, however, due to their greater risk of heart problems.

Almost one in three American adults has high blood pressure, but as there are no blatant symptoms, nearly one-third are undiagnosed, making it a silent killer. In fact, many people have high blood pressure for years without knowing it. The only way to find out is to have your blood pressure checked annually, particularly if you're at higher risk. Age is a definite risk factor for hypertension (about 64 percent of people ages sixty-five to seventy-four have it), along with race (higher incidence in African Americans). Other important risk factors include obesity, diabetes, and a family history of high blood pressure. If you have even one of these, it pays to have your blood pressure checked on a regular basis,

What's more, you should seek early treatment of the condition as soon as you are diagnosed. Undetected or untreated, high blood pressure can cause you to develop some serious health problems over time, such as hardened arteries, heart failure, kidney failure, stroke, or heart attack. Also follow up to make sure that your selected treatment is actually effective. By way of example, one research study reported that only 45 percent of people known to be hypertensive were being treated with medications in 2002, and just 29 percent of them had the condition under control, even though it's well-known that controlling it effectively greatly reduces the risk of all of these potential problems.

Understanding Heart Failure

Each side of your heart is made up of two chambers: the atrium, or upper chamber; and the lower ventricle. Both atria, which are found on the top right and left sides of the heart, receive blood into the heart from either the whole body or the lungs, and the ventricles pump it where it needs to go, out to the lungs or to the entire body. Heart failure occurs when even one of these chambers loses its ability to keep up with pumping out the whole amount of blood coming into it.

Heart failure can involve either side of your heart; however, it usually affects the left side first. If the left ventricle loses its ability to contract normally, this is systolic failure, where the heart can't pump with enough force to push adequate amounts of blood into the circulation. If the ventricle loses its ability to relax normally because the muscle has become stiff, this is diastolic failure, meaning that the heart can't properly fill with blood during the rest period between each beat. Blood coming into the left chamber from the lungs may back up, causing fluid to leak into the lungs, a condition known as pulmonary edema.

As the heart's ability to pump decreases, blood flow slows down everywhere, causing fluid to build up in various tissues, including the lungs. This excess fluid or congestion explains the term *congestive heart failure* used to describe this condition. Left heart failure leads to edema of the lungs, while loss of pumping power on the right side causes blood to back up in veins, resulting in swelling in legs and ankles.

This condition commonly occurs after damage to part of the heart muscle during a heart attack and is associated with a lower quality of life and usually a shortened one. To optimize the rest of your life, particularly if you have already suffered a heart attack, watch out for symptoms of this condition (e.g., shortness of breath or swelling in your lower legs), and talk to your doctor about possibly controlling them with prescribed medications. Heart failure can be treated with varying drugs, including diuretics to drain excess fluids out of the body and others aimed at increasing the pumping power of the heart.

Moderate Your Major Cardiovascular Risk Factors

Major risk factors for cardiovascular problems have been determined (see the sidebar "Major Cardiovascular Risk Factors"). Generally speaking, the more risk factors you have, the greater your chance of developing heart disease or some other form of CVD. Some factors can't be modified, treated, or controlled (e.g., age or sex), while others can. As discussed in the last step, control-

Major Cardiovascular Risk Factors

- Age
- Sex
- Family history of CVD (close male relative younger than fifty-five or close female relative younger than sixty-five)
- Elevated blood fats
- Cigarette smoking
- Hypertension
- Physical inactivity
- Diabetes
- Obesity

ling your level of abdominal obesity usually helps more than worrying about your overall weight. You should also keep in mind that simply having an elevated degree of a particular risk factor increases your overall chances. For example, if your total cholesterol level is 300 milligrams per deciliter (mg/dL), your risk is higher than for someone whose cholesterol runs 245 mg/dL, even though both of you are considered to be in the same high-risk category. Likewise, you can stop or at least reduce cigarette smoking and lower your risk, given that the relative risk of stroke in heavy smokers (more than forty cigarettes a day) is twice that of light smokers (less than ten).

While you can't modify all of your risk factors to protect yourself from future problems, you can certainly take steps to moderate their potential impact on your health and longevity. In the remainder of this step, we discuss some of these risk factors that you can control in more detail and the steps you can easily take to prevent the onset of cardiovascular problems.

Change Your Sex?

Your sex isn't a modifiable risk factor, but a greater knowledge about how it affects your risk will allow you to make informed decisions related to your sex that can somewhat alter your chances of developing CVD. For instance, compared to men, most women are somewhat protected from coronary heart disease, heart attack, and stroke before reaching menopause, which usually occurs in their early fifties. Once women have gone through menopause, their risk begins to rise and keeps rising, making it incorrect to assume that women always have a lower risk and require less aggressive treatment. In reality, within one year after a heart attack, only 62 percent of women compared with 75 percent of men are still living, and more men also survive strokes. Stroke is a leading cause of long-term disability and loss of quality of life for many older females. All types of cardiovascular events are particularly problematic among minority women, especially African Americans. To optimize health and longevity, women can benefit simply by being aware that they likely need to be more aggressive about lowering cardiovascular risk factors after experiencing menopause.

Which Elevated Blood Fats Should Cause Concern?

Cholesterol is a waxy substance made by the liver and also supplied in your diet through animal products, including meats, poultry, fish, shellfish, and dairy products, but it's not found at all in plants. Some cholesterol is needed in your body to insulate nerves, make cell membranes, and produce certain hormones. The total amount of cholesterol in your bloodstream comprises both healthful and harmful types, the majority being high-density lipoproteins (HDL) and low-density lipoproteins (LDL).

HDL is touted as the good type of cholesterol, meaning that it is supposed to protect against heart disease. It has the ability to remove excess cholesterol and may actually take some out of arterial plaques and slow their growth. High levels are associated with a reduced heart attack risk. In fact, low levels of HDL, along with elevated triglycerides (fat), appear to be a stronger predictor of heart-disease-related problems in women than in men. Luckily, you can raise HDL levels and lower triglycerides naturally with increased physical activity. Moderate alcohol consumption, whether it consists of wine, beer, or distilled spirits, apparently cuts the risk of nonfatal heart attacks as well, likely related in part to the beneficial elevations in HDL it causes. Ideally, your HDL levels should be as high as possible. Aim for HDL levels that are higher than 40 mg/dL in men and 50 mg/dL in women for optimal cardiovascular health.

Action Steps for Better Health Tip #43

Your total cholesterol levels don't matter as much as the levels of good and bad types that you have. Small, dense forms of LDL are best lowered, but large, fluffy LDL is relatively benign, while most HDL is beneficial. Have your types and subtypes measured before deciding whether to start taking cholesterol-lowering medications.

Conversely, LDL is considered mostly as the bad type of cholesterol. In particular, oxidation of LDL may contribute most to the development of plaque in coronary and other arteries. A high level of LDL cholesterol (more than 160 mg/dL) reflects an increased risk of heart disease. However, it is now known that there are two types of LDL: a small, dense LDL (sd LDL), which often ends up being taken up into arterial walls and rapidly oxidized, and a large, fluffy LDL that is relatively benign. High levels of the latter type are common in centenarians, while sd LDL is often associated with high triglycerides and heart disease. Thus, sd LDL is the "bad-bad" type of cholesterol, and large, fluffy LDL is the "good-bad" cholesterol. Before being treated for elevated LDL-cholesterol levels, have your doctor measure your levels of both types. If you mainly have the good-bad form, then treatment with medications may not be recommended. You may also ask your doctor to measure your blood levels of lipoprotein (a) and apolipoprotein B, both of which are protein markers for bad-bad cholesterol, to find out more about the types that you have.

Finally, most cholesterol-related recommendations currently suggest that levels be reduced to excessively low values—despite little scientific evidence that doing so is truly beneficial, even for younger individuals. We recommend keeping your LDL at no higher than 120 mg/dL, particularly if you have mostly sd LDL and your HDL levels are less than 70 mg/dL. Aggressively lowering cholesterol levels at ages older than sixty-five, though, should likely be limited to people who have evidence of heart disease, diabetes, or high levels of sd LDL or lipoprotein (a). The drugs of choice for lowering cholesterol levels these days are statins (e.g., Lipitor), which appear to be cardioprotective beyond their lipid-lowering effects by blocking cytokines that damage artery walls and increase plaque formation.

Boost Your Antioxidant Status to Lower Cholesterol's Effects. Antioxidant vitamins—E, C, and beta-carotene, which is a precursor of vitamin A—have potential health-promoting properties. Be careful not to take too much vitamin E, as recent studies have shown that high supplemental doses of vitamin E may actually increase your risk of heart disease. Vitamins consumed naturally through foods are almost always better for you than supplemental ones. So consume more fruits, vegetables, whole grains, and nuts to boost your vitamin E and other vitamin intake. A recent study of the French concluded that each additional fruit or vegetable consumed daily above the minimal recommended intake could cut the risk of heart disease by as much as 4 percent.

Action Steps for Better Health Tip #44

Some easy ways to improve your heart health and lower cholesterol levels through dietary means include eating more fish, drinking moderate amounts of any type of alcohol, eating more vegetables and fruits high in antioxidants, and consuming dark chocolate in limited quantities.

In addition, omega-3 fats found in fish may prevent sudden death or fatal cardiovascular events by regulating heartbeat and preventing irregular rhythms. Cold water fish, such as salmon, tuna, and mackerel, are recommended as good sources of omega-3 fatty acids to be eaten four times a week (as discussed in Step 1). Fish oil supplements at a dose of about 1 gram a day may also reduce the heart rate and normalize heart rhythms in people with and without heart disease.

Likewise, the cacao plant, from which chocolate and cocoa are derived, boosts the immune system and restricts formation of the cholesterol type that damages the coronary vessels. It naturally contains antioxidants called catechins and phenols, as well as over six hundred other plant chemicals. The fat content in dark chocolate comprises equal parts of oleate, a heart-healthy fat also found in olive oil; stearate, which has a neutral effect when eaten in chocolate; and palmitate, which can elevate cholesterol but only comprises one-third of chocolate's fat. Recent studies have indicated that 22 grams of cocoa powder and 16 grams of dark chocolate daily actually can raise HDL cholesterol levels by 10 percent while lowering oxidation of LDL, thereby reducing sd LDL, but milk chocolate may not be nearly as heart healthy, as more of its fat is saturated. Stick with moderate intake of darker types to optimize the workings of your cardiovascular system.

Poorly Controlled Diabetes Causes Heart Disease

Diabetes cases have reached epidemic proportions worldwide and are expected to keep rising during this century. Unfortunately, as far as staying young for longer is concerned, this disease—especially when blood sugars remain poorly controlled—accelerates aging, making the average person with diabetes ten years older biologically than his or her actual chronological age.

By itself, diabetes also constitutes a major risk factor for heart disease and stroke. Older diabetic adults have two to four times the normal risk of suffering from a life-ending heart condition than their nondiabetic peers. Overall, up to 80 percent of people with diabetes die from cardiovascular complications, and their life spans are typically shortened by ten years or more. The statistics are even more disheartening for adults who develop type 2 diabetes at a younger age (by eighteen to forty-four years old): they're fourteen times more likely to have a heart attack, up to thirty times for a stroke.

However, such dismal outcomes are largely preventable by lifestyle choices. Regular physical activity, better food choices, reduced levels of insulin resistance, and more tightly controlled blood glucose levels reduce the risk of developing type 2 diabetes in the first place, help control it more effectively, and lower the chances of ultimately experiencing cardiovascular problems precipitated by it.

Physical Inactivity Decreases Vital Heart Health

Physical activity plays a role in cardiovascular health, given that a sedentary lifestyle in itself increases your risk of all forms of CVD. For instance, less fit people have a 30 to 50 percent greater risk of developing high blood pressure and subsequent strokes, and sedentary people have twice the chance of developing life-shortening heart disease. Regular activity also lowers your risk of developing type 2 diabetes, which by itself is a huge risk factor for CVD.

While regular exercise does not guarantee that you won't get heart disease or other related problems, it can considerably reduce your chances. Doing any physical activity is far better than none, and even low-intensity activities can help prevent heart problems. Refer back to the information about exercise given in Step 2 to get started in being more active to lower your risk of heart attack, stroke, or PVD.

Action Steps for Better Health Tip #45

Remaining sedentary is likely the greatest risk for heart problems that you can have. While regular exercise does not guarantee that you will never experience any heart disease, your chances are far less if you're active. Do both aerobic and resistance work to optimize your insulin action and reduce inflammation.

A Final Word About Step 6

Cardiovascular problems can make you biologically older than your chronological age, thereby reducing your overall health and quality of life. Act immediately to get medical help if you experience any of the usual symptoms of a heart attack or stroke, for the best possible outcome. To stay younger, also take steps to modify or reduce your risk of such events, such as using dietary and exercise interventions to manage high blood pressure, lower blood cholesterol levels, control diabetes, and limit plaque formation in arteries. In addition, you can use medications to control your blood pressure and cholesterol levels, but don't treat your cholesterol levels too aggressively without first checking your subtypes of LDL cholesterol.

Keep Cancer at Bay

"My cancer scare changed my life. I'm grateful for every new healthy day I have. It has helped me prioritize my life."

—*Olivia Newton-John (1948–)*

You'd be hard-pressed to find anyone without some direct exposure to cancer, either through his or her own battle to overcome it or a loved one's struggle. Cancer is second only to cardiovascular problems in causing people in the United States to fail to reach their unique Hayflick limit (the number of times their cells can divide and renew themselves). It is possible to develop cancer at any age. Certain types of this disease—lung, prostate, breast, colorectal, and skin cancer—are more common than others, but they vary by type with regard to how easy they are to treat and how soon you're likely to return to a state of optimal health.

What can you do to protect yourself from getting cancer? Some types can readily be prevented. Lung cancer, the leading cause of cancer-related deaths, is largely preventable with avoidance of cigarette smoking and secondhand smoke inhalation. Risk reduction for certain other cancers is more surprising. For instance, people with diabetes are more likely to develop colon cancer, leaving no doubt that you can lower your risk by achieving more effective control of blood glucose levels; you can also often prevent type

2 diabetes with lifestyle improvements to avoid raising your risk of this cancer at all. To help you stay young for longer, this step discusses the more common types of cancer, what you can do to reduce your risk of developing them, along with how to stay healthier and more vital during medical treatments, if you do have to receive them.

What Causes Cancer and How Widespread Is It?

Cancer results when your own cells start reproducing at a faster rate than normal, usually due to an alteration in the cells' DNA. As you live longer, you'll experience a number of conditions that can increase the odds of getting cancer, such as declines in immune function, longer exposure to potential carcinogens, random gene mutations, a lesser ability to repair bodily injuries, and hormonal changes. Some cancers appear to run in families, but those types usually express themselves when people are younger. It still remains difficult to pinpoint the exact cause of most cancers. Although a diagnosis of cancer is still one of the most dreaded, nowadays cutting-edge advances in medicine allow many types to be treated and completely cured.

This good news needs to be tempered with the fact that the risk of cancer increases with age. People between sixty-five and seventy-four years old have a two- to threefold greater chance of developing it than those between fifty and sixty years old. Cancer is the most common cause of death in people ages sixty to seventy years and the second leading cause in anyone older than eighty. In spite of a fall in its overall incidence in the population as a whole, the fact that the American population is rapidly graying has resulted in an increase in the total number of cases.

Which Cancers Are More Survivable and Common?

Cancer comes in many different forms. Some are relatively benign, such as a slow-growing skin type, while others like pancreatic cancer grow rapidly. Moreover, it can remain localized to one area, or

TABLE 7.1 Number of People Cancer-Free 5 Years After Diagnosis and Treatment (per 100)

	Localized	Local Spread	Distant Spread (Metastatic)
Bladder	92	48	8
Breast (females)	94	73	18
Cervix	90	51	12
Colon	97	60	6
Lung	87	57	9
Pancreas	9	4	2
Prostate (males)	94	85	29
Skin Melanoma	93	57	15
Uterus	94	67	27

it can spread through the blood or lymph system to distant parts of the body. When the latter happens, it is called metastatic. Cancer more commonly spreads via the lymph system, which explains why nearby lymph nodes (e.g., in the armpits for breast tumors) are checked for the presence of abnormal cells as well.

Certain types are more survivable, depending on whether they are localized or spread around the body, as you can see in Table 7.1. In general, the sooner a cancer is diagnosed, the greater your chances of stopping its spread and treating it effectively. Later in this step, you will also learn which screening tests are recommended for early detection and treatment of the more common and easily treatable types.

Lung Cancer. Overwhelmingly, lung cancer is the most common type in anyone older than sixty, followed closely by colorectal. As mentioned, many lung cancer cases could be prevented by avoidance of smoking tobacco products in any form and limited exposure to secondhand smoke. Likewise, if you stop smoking and never start again, you'll lower your risk of developing lung cancer or of having it recur. An increase in antioxidants naturally through intake of more vegetables and fruits may also lower risk.

Colorectal Cancer. Colorectal cancer can affect both the colon, or the large intestine, and the end of the colon, or the rectum. In almost all cases of colorectal cancer, early detection can lead to a cure, making regular screening for anyone older than fifty a must. Its incidence may also be lower in people who eat a low-fat, high-fiber diet, have a limited intake of red meat, and exercise regularly, so adopt these healthier habits to reduce your risk.

Breast Cancer. In women of any age, breast cancer is slightly more common than colorectal. Although younger women certainly can get breast cancer, its incidence in women rises markedly between the ages of sixty-five and eighty-five, and 45 percent of all new cases are diagnosed in women older than sixty-five. Still, that leaves more than half (55 percent) being diagnosed in younger women and also in men. Most breast cancers are located in the upper, outer quadrant of the breast. Other common areas are found under the nipple; in the upper, inner quadrant; and in the lower, inner quadrant. Risk factors include a family history of this cancer, being childless or having children for the first time after age thirty-five, higher intake of animal fats and alcohol, and physical inactivity, among other things. Monthly breast self-exams, along with mammograms (more on these screenings later in this step), may facilitate early detection.

Prostate Cancer. In men, prostate cancer occurs just about as frequently as colorectal. The prostate gland in males is normally about the size and shape of a walnut and is located at the base of the bladder. Its front also surrounds the urethra, the tube that urine flows through. For any American male, the lifetime risk of developing prostate cancer is about 10 percent, although it's rare in men younger than fifty. Older men experience a fortyfold increase in its prevalence between the ages of fifty and eighty-five. It's believed that a high-fat diet may increase your risk of developing this cancer. Some types of prostate cancer are slow-growing and may not become a serious threat to health, but other, more aggressive ones can be.

Prostate cancer often has no symptoms, particularly in the early stages. Symptoms are more likely to occur if and when your cancer grows in the prostate gland and narrows the urethra. Watch out for difficulty in starting to pass urine; a weak, sometimes intermittent flow; dribbling before and after urinating; a frequent or urgent need to urinate; getting up several times in the night to visit the bathroom; (rarely) blood in the urine; and pain during orgasm.

Action Steps for Better Health Tip #46

For a number of reasons, cancer occurs more frequently the older you get. The most common forms of cancer are lung, colorectal, breast (women), prostate (men), and skin, almost all of which are preventable to some degree with dietary improvements, increased physical activity, or other means.

These symptoms are similar to ones produced by a common noncancerous disease called benign prostatic hyperplasia (BPH) where the prostate becomes enlarged. Caused by the multiplication of noncancerous prostate cells, this type of enlargement is very common as well, affecting about half of men in their sixties and up to 90 percent of men in their seventies and eighties. It is less common in men who exercise regularly, though. Luckily, although BPH can cause annoying urinary problems, the presence of prostate gland enlargement is not believed to be directly related to cancer development there.

Skin Cancer. Skin cancers also occur frequently. Worldwide, one in three cancers is skin-related, and among people of all ages, skin cancers currently account for one-half of all cases in the United States. Many are easy to cure if detected early with a thorough skin exam performed by a doctor. Watch for any unusual nodules, lesions, or patches anywhere on your skin; any changes in a mole; or any sores that do not heal, and have them checked out by a doctor. Severe sunburns in childhood and adolescence increase your risk for malignant melanoma, which is much less easily cured and more often a fatal form of skin cancer. Its incidence has purportedly doubled in the past thirty years among Americans, according to the World Health Organization, but you can lower your risk by avoiding tanning salons and by using sunscreens to prevent sunburns.

Is Cancer Different as You Get Older?

Your immune system, particularly the natural killer cells, plays an important role in destroying cancer cells before they can accumulate in your body, and your immune system declines over time, making cancer harder to fight on your own. Loss of telomeres, the ends of chromosomes that control the rate at which cells divide, also occurs as you get older and may play a role in cancer development, along with the body's decreasing ability to repair genetic material found in your DNA.

When it comes down to it, older cells are more prone to developing cancer and when they do become cancerous, they often behave differently. Some cancers, such as breast cancer, actually grow more slowly when you're older. Accordingly, cancer is more likely to respond to hormonal therapy in women older than fifty as there are receptors for estrogen and progesterone in the breast. Certain other types, like acute myelogenous leukemia, respond less well to treatments the older a person gets.

Action Steps for Better Health Tip #47

Even when you're older, as long as you're healthy you should respond as favorably to cancer treatments as anyone younger, so treat it aggressively. Also, try to prevent cancer from occurring through appropriate lifestyle changes like more physical activity, which can work as a preventive therapy even when you're fifty or older.

Can Cancer Be Prevented?

In 1950, smoking was shown to be the number one cause of preventable cancer. Since then, other lifestyle alterations such as the use of sunscreens and increased physical activity have been found to lessen the chances of developing other types, although none is as powerful as smoking cessation's benefit to the lungs. Lifestyle factors with a clear benefit, a probable effect, or a possible one are listed in the sidebar "Lifestyle Factors for Preventing Specific Cancers" along with the cancers most likely prevented (given in parentheses).

Lifestyle Factors for Preventing Specific Cancers

Clear Benefit

- Do not smoke or chew tobacco (lung, oral, esophageal).
- Use sunblock and avoid excessive sun exposure (skin).
- Avoid occupational exposure to cancer-causing toxins or use appropriate protective clothing (skin, lung, and others).
- Increase physical activity (colon and breast).
- Avoid being overweight (colon, breast, and uterine).

Probable Benefit

- Eat more fruits and vegetables (colon, lung, and possibly others).
- Limit intake of red meat (colon).
- Do not consume alcohol excessively (oral, esophageal, breast, and pancreatic).

Possible Benefit*

- Take folic acid and supplements (colon and breast).
- Take selenium supplements (lung, prostate, and colon).
- Take vitamin E supplements (prostate).

*Note that eating a balanced diet with citrus fruit, broccoli, leafy vegetables, asparagus, and tuna most probably is as good as taking these supplemental vitamins and minerals.

Regular Screening Saves Lives

Although there is no evidence yet that early detection reduces men's risk of dying from prostate cancer, regular screenings to detect breast, colon, cervical, and other cancers may in fact increase your chances of surviving them. If you develop any of the symptoms suggestive of cancer or if your risk is higher than average due to family history or other factors, discuss appropriate approaches to screening and diagnosis with your cancer doctor. Symptoms suggestive of cancer include a change in bowel or bladder habits, a sore that does not heal, unusual bleeding or discharge, thickening or a lump in breasts or elsewhere, indigestion or difficulty in swallowing, obvious change in a wart or mole, or a nagging cough or hoarseness.

Action Steps for Better Health Tip #48

Early detection of certain cancers such as breast and colon increases your chances of beating them and remaining healthy for longer. Cancer screenings that are recommended vary with the specific type of cancer, your age, and your unique risk. To determine which screenings to routinely have and the best schedule to follow, consult with your doctor or check the guidelines given by the American Cancer Society at cancer.org.

General screening recommendations are shown in Table 7.2. Currently, there is no recommended screening for lung cancer, although two tools have been developed: chest radiography and sputum cytology. Computerized tomography (CT) screening may be useful for early detection and better survival if you're at high risk for lung cancer (e.g., if you have a history of heavy smoking). Certain screenings have recently become controversial, with debates occurring over the usefulness of breast self-exams and mammography, but they still make sense for the majority of women.

TABLE 7.2 How Often Should You Be Screened for Cancer and How?

	Screening Tool	Before Age 50	After Age 50
Men and Women			
Colorectal	Fecal occult blood test (FOBT) or fecal immunochemical test (FIT)		Annually, for either; for FOBT, use the take-home multiple samples method
	Colonoscopy		Every 10 years, or to follow up on any positive test
Men only			
	Prostate-specific antigen (PSA) and digital rectal exam	Annually starting at age 40 to 45 if high risk, otherwise 50	Annually until 75 years of age
Women only			
Breast	Physician (clinical) breast exam	Every 3 years for ages 20–39, and then annually	Annually
	Self-exam	Optional starting after age 20 (monthly)	Know how breasts feel, and report any changes promptly
	Mammograms	Annually starting at age 40	Annually until at least age 80 if in good health
Cervix	Pap smear	Annually starting 3 years after sexual activity for regular Pap test, or every 2 years using new liquid-based Pap test; go to every 2–3 years at age 30 if normal	Every 2–3 years if smears normal until age 70, but discontinue thereafter unless positive for human papillomavirus

Cancer Therapies Available Today

As far as cancer is concerned, a delay of a few days is unlikely to make a difference to your health, so don't be embarrassed to get a second opinion. If you want to, search for more information on your specific cancer before deciding on which treatment(s) to have. The number of therapies used to treat cancer is constantly increasing, but varies with the type of cancer, its location, and how advanced it is. Therapies commonly employed include surgery, radiation, chemotherapy, hormone therapy, bone marrow transplantation, and biotherapy. Each may be used alone or in conjunction with others, and you may need a combination of two or more for the best outcome in terms of your chances of survival and longevity.

Cancer and most of its therapies cause side effects. A common one is loss of appetite and weight loss, but eating multiple small meals in a day may help. Another is fatigue, but in most cases staying as active as you can and exercising regularly will allow you to maintain function and prevent additional tiredness that results from being out-of-shape physically.

Action Steps for Better Health Tip #49

Commonly used cancer treatments include surgery, radiation, chemotherapy, hormone therapy, bone marrow transplantation, and biotherapy. Each of these therapies may be used alone or in conjunction with others, depending on the type of cancer. If you're unsure about what would be best, research your options and consider getting a second opinion.

Surgical Treatments

Surgery is used for cancers that are localized and easily accessible, such as breast, uterine, cervical, and prostate. It may involve a local incision or require removal of lymph nodes in or near the affected area as well. About 60 percent of cancer patients choose to have surgery, and half of them are cured with this treatment alone. Side effects include pain, infection, fatigue, loss of mobility, and loss of organs or limbs.

Chemotherapy

Chemotherapy is used to treat cancer that has spread (metastasized), or it may be introduced as a secondary line of treatment following surgical removal of a tumor with the goal of treating cancerous areas that may not have been detected on an x-ray or scan. "Chemo" is delivered to all parts of the body through the bloodstream following injection of the drug into a vein or after being taken as a pill by mouth. This therapy is given in repeated cycles of drug delivery followed by recovery periods, so it's not unusual for a course of chemotherapy to take three to nine months. You may experience such side effects as increased risk for infections (fever), low white blood cell count, temporary hair loss, nausea, vomiting, diarrhea, loss of appetite, ulcers of the mouth, candida (a fungal infection), and fatigue. Discuss with your cancer doctor whether you are a candidate for injections that boost white and red blood cells and often decrease the fatigue commonly caused by these treatments.

Radiation

Like surgery, radiation therapy is used for localized cancers that have not spread. More than half of all cancer patients opt to have radiation treatment as part of their therapy, either using a focused, high-energy ray or radioactive implants. The energy ray is painless and is often repeated several times a week over two to three weeks. Be assured that you won't be radioactive or dangerous to other people when receiving this therapy. The implants allow for a more concentrated dose of radiation to be administered to a smaller area for a shorter period of time. They are placed in or near the tumor while you're under local or general anesthesia. Once the implants are surgically removed, no radioactivity remains in the body.

Proton or neutron beam therapy is another specialized form of radiation offered at some cancer centers. If radiation is recommended for you, you should explore whether gamma ray therapy (CyberKnife) may be better for you. It will require going to a specialized center and may not be as convenient to get for that reason.

For all types of radiation, the usual side effects are fatigue, local irritation of the skin, loss of appetite, hair loss at the irradiated site, nausea, vomiting, and diarrhea.

Hormone Therapy

This treatment option involves the use of chemicals that are either naturally produced or that resemble your own hormones. They include corticosteroids, estrogens, progesterone, tamoxifen, and androgens. This therapy often requires the administration of larger doses of hormones than are normally produced by your body and results in side effects that are temporary. Breast cancer in older women is usually more responsive to hormone therapies than when it occurs at a younger age. Mood changes, fluid retention, difficulty sleeping, and osteoporosis are all possible following this therapy.

Immunotherapy

Biotherapy, also called immunotherapy, uses the body's own immune system to fight cancer or to decrease the side effects of other types of cancer treatments. This treatment may interfere with cancer growth, or it may help repair normal cells damaged by other cancer treatments. Drugs such as interleukins, interferons, or tumor necrosis factor are currently being studied in several ongoing clinical trials.

Other Medical Therapies

Alternate medical therapies may be available to treat your cancer, depending on the type. Gene therapy is a promising treatment being studied to determine its usefulness and safety, but it is not used routinely at present. Ask about clinical trials in your area and whether or not you would be eligible to participate.

Alternative Cancer Therapies

Out of desperation, many people seek a variety of alternative therapies or healers after being diagnosed with cancer. While in some areas of medicine alternative therapies are very effective, cancer is not one of them. Numerous alternative therapies are often touted for their ability to cure cancer, but in most cases they're really drugs in disguise and are best avoided. If you're considering one of these alternatives, discuss it with your doctor. If you decide to pursue it, let your doctor know because some of these therapies are extremely toxic and can interact dangerously with any conventional drugs you may already be receiving.

Certain alternative therapies have been shown to be sound, but none of these involves herbs or supplements of any kind. One example of an effective therapy is a positive attitude, which may enhance your body's immune system, thereby decreasing the aggressiveness of your cancer. A positive attitude also makes it easier to cope with the variety of adverse factors that being a cancer patient can bring. Spirituality also can have positive effects; prayer may help the healing process, and religion provides tremendous emotional support. Likewise, exercise increases your circulating levels of beta-endorphins (your body's own morphine-like mood enhancer) and enhances natural killer cells, which are immune cells responsible in part for killing cancer cells. These supportive approaches should not replace appropriate medical therapy, but rather should be considered fellow travelers alongside one another during your journey to become a cancer survivor.

Action Steps for Better Health Tip #50

Sound alternative therapies for cancer don't include herbs or supplements. Instead, try a positive attitude to boost your immune function, spirituality or religion for support, and exercise to raise your feel-good (beta-endorphin) brain hormones, in conjunction with standard medical treatments.

Will Your Cancer Come Back?

There is no standard of care yet about how often you should be rescreened if you have already had cancer. In the absence of any guidelines, you should likely be screened every three months for two years afterward for returning signs of your cancer. The goal of this increased surveillance is to find the cancer before the symptoms return. This increased rate of screening applies only to the specific type of cancer you had. If the cancer does not return within two years, then the schedule for screening is reduced over the next few years to the frequency recommended for people who never had it.

A Final Word About Step 7

A diagnosis of cancer, although frightening, is not a reason to lose hope. Instead, it is a time to explore options and make a plan to get the best care you can. The more allies you have on your road to recovery, the more likely you are to survive the cancer and thrive afterward. Some cancers appear to run in families, but those types usually express themselves when people are young. Other types are preventable through lifestyle choices. The single greatest risk factor for getting cancer is aging. The older you become, the greater your chances of getting this disease for myriad reasons. Whatever the cause, the importance of early detection through screening and quick treatment following detection, after considering all of your treatment options, can't be overemphasized.

Thicken Up Your Bones

"Old age must be resisted and its deficiencies supplied."
—*Cicero (106–43* B.C.*)*

"It is the soundness of the bones that ultimates itself in a peach-bloom complexion."
—*Ralph Waldo Emerson (1803–1882)*
in Conduct of Life (VIII: Beauty)

Healthy bones and joints are crucial to your mobility and extended youthfulness, as well as to living a pain-free life as you move around. Some largely effective strategies exist to prevent and limit potential bone problems, no matter what your age is, including adequate calcium and vitamin D intake, regular weight-bearing exercises, avoidance of phosphorus-filled sodas, moderation of protein intake, and in some cases hormone replacement therapies. All of these options for improving bone health are addressed in this step, along with how to maintain healthy joints in order to reduce and minimize pain from any arthritis you may develop, to help you stay feeling younger than your chronological age.

Thinning Bones: Risk, Screening, Prevention, and Treatment

Unfortunately, everyone is experiencing slow bone demineralization throughout adulthood starting around the age of twenty-five, which can eventually lead to fractures and a lower quality of health. This process, known as osteoporosis, can lead to a greater incidence of fractures, especially of your hip, wrist, or spine, at whatever age you finally reach a critical minimum bone density. According to the National Osteoporosis Foundation, 50 percent of women and 25 percent of men over fifty will have an osteoporotic fracture in their lifetime. Moreover, the surgeon general's report issued in 2004 predicted that by 2020 half of all Americans ages fifty and older will have weak bones if there are no significant changes to the nation's diet and lifestyle as a whole. At present, an estimated 10 million Americans—80 percent of them female—already have this disease, and another 34 million have significantly reduced bone mass (a condition known as osteopenia). Thinning bones is not a problem to ignore if you want to live long and well.

The term *osteoporosis* was originally coined in the early nineteenth century, but it wasn't until 1940 that the loss of estrogen in women at menopause was identified as playing a role in its development. It has often been asserted that osteoporosis is actually a pediatric disease because the amount of calcium you ingest during your childhood likely is a major determinant of your bone mineral density later in life. Regardless of when it actually starts, it's undeniably a chronic condition that causes bones to gradually lose their stored calcium, leaving them porous and brittle. Over time, this process of demineralization causes the skeleton to become weaker, and when it reaches a critically low level, bone fractures can occur and recur from seemingly minor impacts.

Whereas bone loss occurs over many years, you will likely only become aware of having this condition when fractures are blatant or postural changes are well advanced. For example, repeated, undetected compression fractures in the vertebrae of the spine can lead to stooped posture and backaches, both of which are common characteristics of older women (and some men). Hip fractures resulting from this disease can be immensely debilitating, often signaling the start of a downward trend of reduced strength and a lower quality of life.

Action Steps for Better Health Tip #51

Risk factors for osteoporosis include advancing age, female sex, early menopause, hereditary factors, small frame size, and more. Take steps to lower your risk from other contributing factors by not smoking, consuming alcohol only moderately, engaging in regular physical activity, and taking in adequate calcium and vitamin D.

Who Is at Risk for Osteoporosis?

Certain immutable factors increase your risk of developing osteoporosis. Among them are small frame size, female sex, age, hereditary factors, Caucasian or Asian race, early menopause, prolonged immobilization, low levels of estrogen or testosterone, excess thyroid hormones (e.g., overactive thyroid gland), and extended steroid use (such as prednisone). Other contributory behaviors like cigarette smoking, excessive alcohol consumption, physical inactivity, and inadequate intake of calcium and vitamin D can be controlled and modified to lower risk.

Women have an inherently greater risk for osteoporosis than men not only because men's skeletons contain a larger reserve of bone minerals but also due to faster rates of loss in females. After menopause, women lose bone at an average rate of 2 to 3 percent per year, while men of a similar age are losing only 0.4 percent annually. The most visible sign of this bone loss is a gradual shortening in overall height over time. In Caucasian and Asian women in particular, bone mass starts to decrease in the femur (thigh bone) in their midtwenties, followed by spine losses in their mid- to late-thirties, and arm bone demineralization after forty years of age.

Screening for Osteoporosis

Due to recent advances in the way bone density is measured, it's now easier than ever to find out if you already have significant bone loss, if you're preosteoporotic (i.e., you have osteopenia), or even if you're at risk for osteoporosis in the future. Testing methods include single–photon absorptiometry (SPA), dual–photon absorptiometry (DPA), dual–energy x–ray absorptiometry (DXA), computed tomography (CT) scanning, and ultrasound. If you have already suffered a bone fracture of the wrist, back, or hip seen on x–ray, you don't need to have a special test done before being treated for osteoporosis; it's assumed that you already have it.

All women reaching the age of menopause should have their bone mineral density measured, along with at least one more check at sixty–five years of age. Since they lag behind, men should ideally have testing done when they reach sixty–five to seventy years old. The actual diagnosis of osteoporosis is made when you have a bone mineral density that is more than 2.5 standard deviations below the young–adult average (a T score of 1 to 2.5). Your bone mineral density should be repeated after two years to determine your rate of bone loss, and the testing should always be repeated at the same time of year, as seasonal changes in bone density are common.

Action Steps for Better Health Tip #52

Screening for osteoporosis is important for preventing problems. Women should have their bone mineral density measured at menopause and at least once more at sixty-five years of age. Men should be tested when they reach sixty-five to seventy years old. If you have a fracture of your wrist, spine, or hip seen on an x-ray, you should be treated for osteoporosis.

Prevent Bone Loss and Strengthen Your Bones

The best preventive measure is to start out with the highest peak bone mineral density that you possibly can in your midtwenties.

The rate of loss of bone minerals is fairly steady over time, so having denser bones at your peak allows you to live longer without reaching a critical osteoporotic fracture level. Preventive strategies include appropriate exercise, adequate calcium intake, dietary modifications, and boosting vitamin D levels. You can also take steps now to improve your current bone health, even if the process can't be completely reversed. Finally, you may want to consider hormone replacement therapies or other medications to ensure that your bones stay healthy throughout your lifetime.

Action Steps for Better Health Tip #53

To prevent osteoporosis, start out with the highest peak bone mineral density that you can in your midtwenties. If you missed out on this opportunity, focus now on a regular program of moderate, weight-bearing exercise; resistance workouts; adequate calcium and vitamin D intake; and medications (including possible estrogen or testosterone replacement, if recommended by your physician).

Appropriate Exercise for Bone Health. Whether or not you have osteoporosis, it's advisable for you to begin a program of moderate, weight-bearing exercise, especially if you don't already exercise regularly. These exercises include walking and aerobics, and they strengthen bone while increasing bone-forming processes. In addition, most types of resistance or weight training positively stress bones and result in calcium phosphate deposition, resulting in thicker, healthier bones. Studies on women with significant osteoporosis engaging in resistance training for a year have shown a small, but measurable, increase in bone mineral density; conversely, their similarly aged, nonexercising peers experienced a decline in their bone thickness over the same time period. So even if you can't completely reverse the thinning process, you can certainly slow it down significantly or even stop it in its tracks for a time.

Taking in Enough Calcium. Women in the United States consume an average of only 500 milligrams of calcium per day, which is less than half the recommended daily allowance for younger adults. Adequate calcium intake from childhood through your midthirties is crucial to the development of the greatest possible deposits of calcium phosphate salts in bone. It's less certain whether adding calcium to your diet after menopause can prevent bone loss; however, women who consume large amounts of calcium experience fewer hip fractures. Most doctors recommend that adult women and men consume between 1,000 and 1,200 milligrams of calcium per day, with the higher intake recommended for postmenopausal women older than fifty and not taking estrogen and everyone older than sixty-five.

Calcium supplements are certainly one way to ensure adequate intake, but it can also be accomplished through intake of calcium-rich foods (Table 8.1), which is the preferred method, as doing so through your diet can convey other health benefits as well. According to most nutritionists, the best choices are low- or non-fat dairy products. If you avoid milk because of lactose intolerance, the most reliable way to get calcium is to choose lactose-reduced or low-lactose alternative dairy products, such as cheese, yogurt, or lactase-treated milk, or to consume the enzyme lactase before consuming milk products to aid digestion.

On the other hand, others and particularly vegans (complete vegetarians) would argue that many green vegetables have calcium absorption rates of more than 50 percent, compared with about 32 percent for milk, making vegetables potentially a better source. A recent article in the *American Journal of Clinical Nutrition* reported calcium absorption to be about 53 percent for broccoli, 64 percent for brussels sprouts, 58 percent for mustard greens, 52 percent for turnip greens, and 40 to 59 percent for kale. Likewise, beans (e.g., pinto beans, black-eyed peas, and navy beans) and bean products, such as tofu, are rich in calcium. About 36 to 38 percent of the calcium in calcium-fortified orange juice is absorbed (as reported by manufacturer's data). Even most fruits contain some calcium,

TABLE 8.1 Food Sources and Absorption Rates of Calcium

Food Source	Calcium Content (mg)	Fractional Absorption (%)
Cow's milk, 1 cup	250–300	32
Most cheeses, 1.5 oz.	305–336	32
Yogurt, low-fat, 8 oz. container	338–448	32
Soy milk, calcium-fortified, 1 cup	75–300	24
Tofu, medium or firm, ½ cup	130 (medium), 258 (firm)	31
Pink salmon, canned, with bone, 3 oz.	181	27
Sardines, Atlantic, in oil, drained, 3 oz.	325	27
Rainbow trout, farmed, cooked, 3 oz.	173	27
Ocean perch, Atlantic, cooked, 3 oz.	116	27
Most canned beans, 1 cup	69–161	17
Turnip greens, boiled, 1 cup	198	52
Chinese cabbage (bok choy), boiled, 1 cup	158	54
Spinach, boiled, 1 cup	244	5
Kale, boiled, 1 cup	94	59
Mustard greens, boiled, 1 cup	82	58
Broccoli, boiled, 1 cup	178	53
Brussels sprouts, boiled, 1 cup	56	64
Cauliflower, boiled, 1 cup	34	69
Navel orange, 1 medium	56	N/A
Orange juice, calcium-fortified, 1 cup	300	25
Almonds, dry roasted, 1 cup	80	21

albeit relatively small amounts, as do most nuts and seeds. The amount of calcium that can be absorbed from these foods varies, so both calcium content and its bioavailability, shown in Table 8.1, should be considered. Some plant foods have calcium that is well absorbed but low in total content per serving.

Many green leafy vegetables, beans, calcium-fortified soy milk, and calcium-fortified 100 percent juices are equally good, and some are even superior calcium sources with advantages that dairy products lack. These alternate foods are excellent sources of phytochemicals and antioxidants, while containing little fat, no cholesterol, and no animal proteins, which in excess can actually cause the loss of calcium from bones.

Action Steps for Better Health Tip #54

For optimal absorption of calcium from foods, consider consuming more green leafy vegetables, beans, calcium-fortified soy milk, and calcium-fortified 100 percent juices, not just dairy products. Check the calcium content and bioavailability as they can vary.

Can Too Much Calcium Be Bad? In general, calcium absorption decreases as your intake goes up, thereby providing a protective mechanism to lessen the chances of absorbing too much. An intake of about 4 grams (4,000 mg) per day, however, can lead to calcium toxicity, with high blood calcium levels, severe kidney damage, and calcium deposition, or milk-alkali syndrome. This syndrome occurs most often as a result of antacid abuse, which results in excessive calcium carbonate intake. Supplementing with up to 1,500 mg of calcium per day appears to be safe, but use caution if you have a history of kidney stones. Excess calcium can increase its excretion in urine, which increases the risk of kidney stone formation. In addition, taking in too much calcium without adequate fluid intake can lead to constipation.

Moderating Your Diet in Other Important Ways. Calcium aside, bone mineral loss can be affected by your intake of other foods and beverages. For instance, phosphorus–filled sodas (dark colas) are unhealthy for your bones for two reasons: (1) they contain high amounts of phosphoric acid, which can cause an imbalance between blood levels of calcium and phosphorus, resulting in calcium loss from bones; and (2) caffeine added in most sodas can additionally mobilize bone calcium. Ideally, your dietary intake of calcium and phosphate should be balanced equally (1:1), but many people consume up to fifteen times more phosphate, as it is widely distributed in foods and beverages.

The real issue is that a calcium-phosphate imbalance triggers the release of parathyroid, a hormone that causes your bones to release more calcium into your bloodstream and a loss of bone density when excess phosphates are consumed over a lifetime. High phosphorus intake may also accelerate the ability of elevated blood glucose levels to damage your body through the formation of advanced glycation end products (AGEs) that cause premature aging. Thus, there are many good reasons for drinking very limited amounts of phosphate-containing sodas.

Action Steps for Better Health Tip #55

Other compounds found in food and drinks can affect your bones as well. For optimal bone health, severely limit your intake of phosphorus-containing colas, caffeine, animal protein, and sodium.

Even higher intakes of protein may increase your bone mineral loss. The effect of excess protein intake on bone health remains unclear, but some studies show that diets that are high protein, especially in animal protein, cause increased losses of calcium in the urine and may even increase fracture risk. These effects may be especially important if your calcium intake is marginal or low. Other studies, however, suggest that a higher protein intake is needed to promote calcium absorption, reduce the risk of fracture, and increase bone density. Until further evidence is available, it would be best for you to meet recommended calcium intakes and to consume adequate (at least 1.2 grams of protein per kilogram of body weight daily to maintain muscle mass), but not excessive, amounts of protein from nonplant sources.

Finally, a final dietary factor in bone health is total sodium intake. Sodium increases calcium losses, with an estimated 5 to 10 milligrams of calcium lost with each gram of salt eaten. It is likely that reducing your sodium intake can positively impact your bone mineral content. In general, diets like Atkins that are high in protein and often in sodium actually contribute to osteoporosis and are best avoided for the long term, if for no other reason than this.

Taking in Enough Vitamin D for Healthy Bones. As discussed in Step 3, it's vitally important to get enough vitamin D, which helps the body absorb calcium, particularly for men older than sixty-five and women older than fifty. As you get older, your skin manufactures less vitamin D in response to ultraviolet (UV) rays, so obtaining five to fifteen minutes of sunlight exposure each day may not be adequate even though it was when you were younger. As this vitamin is fat soluble, you can also find it in fish liver oils such as cod liver oil, liver, and egg yolks. In addition, margarine, milk, and cereals are often fortified with it.

Since it's still unlikely that sunlight and food alone will provide sufficient amounts as you get older, you likely will need to supplement with vitamin D. For adults younger than fifty, the usual recommended daily intake is 200 international units (IU), which doubles to 400 IU once you reach fifty. The potential youthful effects of having enough of this vitamin are usually underestimated, so we (and others) recommend 800 IU as an optimal daily dose for anyone fifty and older.

Hormones and Bone Health

It is well established that estrogen is essential for the maintenance of normal bone minerals. Despite the recent controversy from the Women's Health Initiative, women experiencing early menopause should consider taking supplemental estrogen for bone health at least until the age that most women go through menopause, about fifty-two years. In addition, women with low bone minerals and a normal menopausal age should take estrogen, and in some cases progesterone, for five years after menopause, but not after age sixty. Appropriate estrogen dosing is discussed in Step 3.

As for testosterone, it appears that this androgenic hormone may stimulate bone formation, while estrogen only prevents its loss. Males with low testosterone levels may need to take this hormone to protect their bones, and it may also improve bone strength in women. A medication called Livial is a unique estrogen-progesterone-testosterone agent that may be particularly useful for some women to reduce hot flashes and improve bone mineral content. Not available in the United States, it is currently sold in the rest of the world.

Action Steps for Better Health Tip #56

If your bones are thinning excessively, consider hormone therapy using estrogen, testosterone replacement, or both. In addition, your bone health can be improved by use of other medications such as Fosamax, Actonel, Boniva, Evista, and calcitonin.

Treating Osteoporosis with Other Medications

In addition to making healthy dietary and other lifestyle changes to improve your bone health, you may also need to consider using prescribed medications that can enhance bone mineral content. Drugs for treating osteoporosis include bisphosphonates (Fosamax, Actonel, and Boniva), raloxifene (Evista), calcitonin, and parathyroid hormone analogs. The first two classes of drugs are taken by mouth. Calcitonin is a naturally occurring hormone produced by your parathyroid gland, but a synthetic form is available as a nasal spray. Similarly, an analog of parathyroid hormones given by injection can help stimulate your bones to get stronger. Some other new drugs are in the pipeline and include medications that may work as antibodies to your body's natural hormones that cause bone thinning.

At present, most women and men who have or are at risk for thinning bones should at least take a bisphosphonate, along with supplemental calcium and vitamin D for at least five years. A controversy exists over whether taking bisphosphonates for longer may actually lead to the development of more brittle bones. If you have been taking them for longer than this time frame, you should discuss with your doctor whether to continue their use.

Maintain Optimal Joint Health

Arthritis is the painful inflammation of a joint or joints, and having to live with the daily pain can make you feel a lot less youthful. The most common type is osteoarthritis caused by degeneration of bony joint surfaces, usually in the knees, hips, spine, hands, and toes. Often described as "wear and tear" arthritis, it affects more than 15 million Americans and is more common in joints that have been previously injured, particularly traumatically, such as through contact sports. In addition, lower extremity joints are more likely to become arthritic if you're overweight, since carrying around more weight puts additional stress on cartilage in hip and knee joints.

Action Steps for Better Health Tip #57

You may have arthritis in your joints if you experience pain (especially made worse by cool, damp weather), crackling or popping (mostly in knees), swelling, stiffness, and restrictions, instability, or "locking up" with movement. Check with your doctor if you have any of these symptoms to come up with an effective treatment plan.

What Causes Arthritis?

Arthritis can result from trauma or from repetitive use, although often no single cause is identifiable. Joints, formed by the juxtaposition of two or more bones with cartilage coating on their ends, normally function to provide flexibility, stability, support, and protection to the skeleton, enabling movement of limbs. In a healthy joint, this coating maintains the separation between bones, allowing joints to move smoothly and without pain. In the early stages of this type of arthritis, the cartilage's surface becomes swollen (inflamed), forming tiny crevasses that hinder movement. A loss of elasticity in the cartilage also makes it more vulnerable to further damage, and outgrowths known as bone spurs often begin to form around its edges. Other associated joint structures, such as the synovial fluid in the middle of joints, tendons, and ligaments, can also become inflamed. In advanced cases, the cartilage cushion is completely lost, limiting joint mobility.

How Can You Tell if You Have Arthritis?

Arthritis is easily identifiable by the symptoms listed in the sidebar "Symptoms of Arthritis," although their degree varies widely among individuals. It can cause pain in the affected joint or joints after repeated use, especially later in the day, or you may experience swelling, pain, and stiffness after long periods of inactivity (e.g., after sleep or sitting for a long time) that subsides with activity.

Symptoms also vary with the affected joint. For instance, if you have knee arthritis, you may experience problems with that joint locking up, especially when stepping up or down. Hip problems usually make you limp, while affected finger joints often result in reduced strength and movement, making simple tasks such as buttoning clothes or opening jars difficult. Affected finger joints can also result in hard, bony enlargements. An arthritic spine can cause neck and low back pain, along with weakness and numbness, particularly if you have developed bony spurs there.

Symptoms of Arthritis

- Pain, made worse by cool, damp weather
- Crackling or popping in the affected joints (most commonly knees)
- Enlarged, swollen joints, often tender when touched
- Stiffness and restricted movement in affected joints
- Unstable joints that move too far or in the wrong direction

The pain that you feel doesn't come from the joint cartilage surfaces themselves, as they contain no nerve endings, but rather from the irritated nerves in adjacent stretched or inflamed areas. You can also experience what is known as "referred pain," meaning that you feel it somewhere other than in the affected joint. For example, an arthritic spine can cause pain in your neck, arms, or legs. Pain is only continuous when almost all of the cartilage surfaces of joints have been eroded, at which point it is indicative of advanced arthritis.

Will Exercise Help or Hurt My Joints?

To prevent painful flare-ups, avoid doing intense activities that can further injure the joint's bony surfaces. Moderate aerobic exercise can be beneficial as long as it is performed at an intensity that is not injurious. For example, even a six-month weight-loss and walking program has been shown to result in lesser arthritic pain in overweight and obese postmenopausal women with knee arthritis. Vigorous running, however, would likely further damage such knee joints.

To further protect arthritic joints, focus on strengthening surrounding muscles that support and protect them. For instance, for your knees, work on strengthening both groups of muscles in your thigh that affect knee movement, including your quadriceps in the front (knee extensors) and hamstrings in the back of your thigh (flexors). In addition, non–weight-bearing ones like stationary cycling, aquatic activities, and light to moderate resistance work that put lower amounts of stress on joints should result in less pain and fewer arthritis–related problems.

Action Steps for Better Health Tip #58

Regular moderate aerobic activity will improve symptoms of arthritis, as long as the chosen exercise is not overly stressful to affected joints. Switching to non-weight-bearing activities like cycling and aquatic exercise may also help, along with engaging in strength and full range-of-movement exercises for painful joints.

Treatment of Arthritis

Much of the treatment for arthritis involves no prescriptions at all, focusing instead on ways to relieve painful joints through more practical changes or treatments. Try any or all of the suggestions given in the sidebar "Nonmedication Treatments of Arthritic Pain" that pertain to your affected joints to help prevent and alleviate pain without the need for additional medications.

Medications to Manage Arthritic Pain. If you need additional relief, prescription and nonprescription drugs are also available to help alleviate your pain. Your best bet is to start with an over-the-counter pain reliever, such as acetaminophen (Tylenol). If this medication doesn't work, try taking nonsteroidal anti-inflammatory drugs (NSAIDs) such as Advil and Nuprin, Aleve, or aspirin in recommended doses. The main problem with NSAIDs is that they can

Nonmedication Treatments of Arthritic Pain

- Participate in regular, moderate aerobic exercise.
- Perform strengthening and full range-of-motion exercises for painful joints.
- Receive massage therapy on muscles surrounding affected joints.
- Use heat and cold packs whenever pain is bothersome and after exercise.
- Use special gadgets to open jars to reduce stress on finger joints.
- Use athletic tape around an arthritic knee to support and stabilize it.
- Wear wedged insoles in your shoes for hip or knee problems (or orthotics, particularly if you have one leg longer than the other).
- Lose weight, primarily through exercise, to alleviate lower extremity arthritis pain.
- Use a cane or walking stick with painful hips or knees.

cause stomach problems and kidney damage over time, and if you already have pain from arthritis, you will likely need to use these drugs for many years.

For painkillers to work effectively, you must take them regularly, not just when you can no longer stand the pain. It's particularly important to take a dose before going to bed so that you don't wake up stiff and sore the next morning, particularly after a day when you have been more active than usual.

In rare cases of extreme pain, you can ask your physician to prescribe stronger pain medications, but be aware that they can be addictive and must be used with caution. Moreover, at least one anti-inflammatory prescription pain medication, Vioxx, was recently taken off the market due to concerns that it minimally doubled the risk of heart attacks and stroke compared with older, nonprescription pain medications such as Aleve. A mechanistically similar drug, Celebrex, is still available by prescription, however.

Keep in mind that any medications you take to control your pain, even over-the-counter ones, have the potential to interact with drugs that you may be taking for other health problems. Always be certain to let your doctor know what medicines you're taking, so that appropriate dosing and scheduling of all of your drugs can be coordinated.

Dietary and Herbal Remedies. Dietary changes that can alleviate inflammation may help reduce arthritic pain, although many of these remedies remain unproven. For example, some research has shown that foods rich in omega-3 fatty acids (e.g., fish and walnuts) and the spices ginger and turmeric may help reduce inflammation, while antioxidant-rich plant foods can potentially help reduce tissue damage from inflammation. You may benefit by adding oily fish and other sources of omega-3 fatty acids, along with plenty of antioxidant-rich vegetables and fruits, to your daily diet.

The jury is still out on herbal remedies, such as supplementing with glucosamine sulfate and chondroitin, two natural treatments for arthritis, but the latest research doesn't look too promising. In addition, certain natural herbs and spices, such as ginger, holy basil, turmeric, green tea, rosemary, scutellaria, and huzhang, are thought to contain naturally occurring anti–inflammatory compounds known as COX-2 inhibitors, which are also found in the prescription drug Celebrex and previously Vioxx. The benefit of any of these dietary supplements for arthritic pain has yet to be proven with scientific trials.

Action Steps for Better Health Tip #59

Try nonmedicinal methods such as exercise, massage, and others to alleviate pain from arthritis, followed by pain relievers and anti-inflammatory drugs (e.g., Tylenol, Advil, Aleve, and Celebrex). Don't be afraid of having surgery when you can no longer control the pain and it's interfering with your daily functioning.

Do You Have to Have Surgery?

If you reach the point where your pain is severe and joint function is inadequate due to your arthritis, seriously consider having surgery. While this option previously was only a last resort, it's now becoming an earlier, effective option for treating chronic arthritic pain, particularly of the knee. Many types of surgical procedures are available to treat different joints, with the most well-known being artificial joint replacement for completely destroyed joints. Other less dramatic surgical procedures may treat arthritis in early stages and slow the progression of the disease, however. The good news is that this condition doesn't always worsen over time. You may find that your symptoms stabilize, and even if the arthritis progresses, it may do so very slowly, giving you plenty of time to explore other options.

Technological advances in materials, operative procedures, product design and manufacturing processes have brought joint replacement surgeries into the new millennium with a flourish. Surgical techniques are becoming more successful every day due to new bone substitutes, specialized alloys, and innovative designs for replacement joints. In the near future, you may be able to look forward to minimally invasive joint replacement surgeries and more—so stay tuned.

A Final Word About Step 8

Osteoporosis, or thinning bones, can result in fractures that can severely limit your ability to function and quality of life. The good news is that this disease is largely preventable with adequate amounts of calcium and vitamin D, participation in regular weight-bearing exercise like walking or resistance training, dietary improvements, and hormone replacement therapies. Pain from arthritis can also greatly lower how good you feel, but it can be effectively controlled through a variety of nonmedicinal and medicinal means, including exercise, dietary changes, pain relievers, anti-inflammatory drugs, and surgical options, that can help you feel more youthful for longer.

Remain on Your Feet

"Teach us to live that we may dread unnecessary time in bed. Get people up and we may save our patients from an early grave."
—*Dr. Richard Alan John Asher (1912–1969)*

This next-to-last step in your journey focuses specifically on prevention of falls and frailty, both of which become more common the older you get. Nowadays, almost everyone is aware of the potential for bad falls and the consequent need for medical assistance. TV commercials for LifeCall's medical alarm systems that started airing in 1989 raised this awareness. They depicted wearable devices that a prostrate elderly individual could use to call for emergency medical services (EMS) by pushing a button and saying into it, "I've fallen and I can't get up." Their ads had the effect of turning this common and potentially fatal situation into a joke represented by this catchphrase that has become a universal punch line for comedians. It hasn't lost its universal appeal yet. A remarkably similar phrase—"Help, I've fallen and I can't get up!"—became a registered trademark of Life Alert Emergency Response, Inc., in 2002.

Actually, it's no laughing matter. Everyone falls down at one time or another, even if it's just because you accidentally trip over your own feet. Even if you have been fortunate enough to stay on your feet or to not become injured from a fall, there's no guarantee that your good fortune will continue as you reach and pass the sixty-year milestone, particularly if you're a younger woman with osteoporosis or osteopenia. If you ever experience a hip fracture related to falling down, you may not be able to get up on your own. Other individuals simply lack the strength or agility to do so, particularly if they have suffered from significant muscle wasting over a period of time.

Admittedly, no one likes to consider the possibility of reaching a physical state that would not allow independent living, but both falls and frailty can make this a reality. Even fewer of us want to end up living out the rest of our lives in a nursing home, away from our family and friends and cared for by relative strangers. Even if you're still feeling young and good enough to not have to worry about these possible scenarios yet, you may have parents or older relatives who are being affected. It's better to know which path to follow to prevent such scenarios altogether as time inevitably marches on, which is the real goal of discussing them in this step.

Falls: Impact and Prevention

Falling down occasionally is inevitable at any age. In fact, the more active you are, the more likely you are to fall down at some point, even if you're in good shape and have excellent balance. Despite what you might suspect about falls being associated with getting out of the house, most of them actually occur indoors, mainly in the bathroom, bedroom, and kitchen. Ten percent of falls occur on the stairs, particularly during descent, with the first and last steps being the most dangerous. Therefore, it is essential for you to set goals designed to minimize the impact of falls—both the number and the potential injuries—rather than to ineffectively attempt to lower the risk of falling by becoming more physically inactive, which would be extremely counterproductive.

The potentially negative impact of falling down is undeniable. About 95 percent of all hip fractures result from falls and are the major cause of hospital emergency room visits for injuries; they account for more than 800,000 emergency room visits and more than 332,000 hospital admissions each year. In addition, the psychological aspects can be equally damaging. Fear of falling, which may cause individuals to choose to become less active and less social, can lead to isolation, depression, and impaired activities of daily living due to further declines in strength. Although falls are less common among adults in their middle years, one in three people older than sixty falls each year, so they are a serious problem.

What Are the Primary Risk Factors for Falling?

The major risk factors associated with falls are quadriceps (thigh muscle) weakness, balance problems, gait disorders, sensory loss, dizziness, recent changes in medication(s), upright posture, ill-fitting glasses or new bifocals that affect downward vision, and a history of falls. The risk factors can be remembered with the SAFE AND SOUND mnemonic shown in the sidebar on the next page.

Action Steps for Better Health Tip #60

Falls are inevitable, regardless of what age you are. Some major risk factors include muscular weakness, poor vision, medication effects, unsteady balance, and getting up to urinate frequently at night. Minimize the potential impact of falls by keeping yourself healthy, strong, stable, and physically active, particularly focusing on daily balance and strength exercises.

Other risks arise from how well you are, or aren't. For example, your risk of falling is higher whenever you develop a new disease or condition that significantly impacts your health, even if it only has a temporary effect. Fainting for any reason (e.g., due to a drop in blood pressure after eating, abnormal heart rhythms, anemia, straining while urinating or defecating, and use of certain medications) causes you to rapidly "get horizontal." Delirium is its own risk factor for falls, and it often accompanies the onset of a new disease as well. Dementia doubles the risk compared to mentally healthier counterparts. For anyone with Alzheimer's disease, fall

Risk Factors for Falling at Any Age

Strength problems (particularly in quadriceps muscles)

Alcohol in excess

Food-associated low blood pressure

Environmental factors (such as uneven surfaces or poor lighting)

Atherosclerotic disease (fainting)

No freedom (restraints that keep you from being physically active)

Drugs (medication effects)

Sight problems (poor vision from cataracts, glaucoma, or macular degeneration)

Orthostasis (dizziness or disorientation with standing)

Unsteady balance

Nocturia (a frequent need to urinate during the night)

Delirium

risk is increased due to taking shorter steps, swaying more, and varying gait from one step to the next.

How frequently or urgently you have to go to the bathroom also, strangely enough, affects your falling risk. As mentioned, making frequent trips to urinate at night (nocturia) sets you up to fall, as can incontinence at any time of day. If you're rushing to make it to the bathroom in time, you're more likely to fall due to your altered gait and abnormally rapid pace. Poorer lighting also increases the risk of falling when you get up during the night. You should keep your feet in good shape, too, because bunions, calluses, and deformed toes can modify gait or inhibit adequate movement, thus heightening your fall risk, and you should forget wearing wobbly high-heel shoes if you want to stay on your feet.

What's more, getting older by itself is associated with a number of physical changes that increase your risk of falling, such as having a more variable gait and a slower walking speed. In particular, your gait may become more unstable when you're focusing on doing something else while walking. Combine that with less flexible ankles and weaker legs, and you have a recipe for disaster. Trying to stand on your tiptoes can also increase your instability. You tend to lose strength in the muscles on the sides of your thighs (lateral quadriceps), and if you already have trouble walking sideways like a crab, your risk of falling down when moving around is much greater. Finally, unless you work hard to maintain it, your balance can become poorer over time, possibly resulting in increased falls.

Preventing Falls

Many of the potential risks arising from physical changes as you get older can be substantially lowered by doing strengthening, balance, and flexibility exercises (found in Step 2). Furthermore, you can prevent falls by properly lighting areas where you're walking, particularly at night; wearing good shoes; correcting your vision (e.g., cataract removal); resting when you get tired; controlling incontinence with medications or other means; and removing floor clutter and throw rugs.

Not leaving things on the floor that you could trip over may seem like a given, but both of us know reasonably young individuals (well under fifty years of age) who have tripped and fallen over items that they left in unexpected places on the floor. In one case, a woman whom Dr. Sheri knew tripped over some clothes she had left on the floor. She had osteopenia, the precursor to osteoporosis, and she suffered a longitudinal fracture of the upper arm bone (humerus). Besides being quite painful, this fracture also required months of immobilization to heal properly, causing her to go on disability leave from her work for over four months. Finally, if

193

you're prone to falling frequently, you may also want to look into wearing hip pads to soften your landings and lower the potential for hip fractures.

Frailty: The Beginning of the End?

Frailty generally marks the end of an independent lifestyle for an older population, but luckily it is largely preventable. People who become frail undeniably experience a decline in their mobility. As a consequence, they usually are less socially active, fall down more, are more prone to fractures due to osteoporosis, may become incontinent, and lose much of their quality of life. In fact, falls can be an important marker of frailty, particularly because they frequently play a role in accelerating the loss of health and independence of a frail individual and can lead to decreased activity, depression, social isolation, functional decline, and a diminished quality of life. Moreover, a fear of falling that keeps them from being active only makes their ability to function on any level decline faster. All in all, becoming frail is not a pretty picture!

A Definition of Frailty

Frailty has been defined by some as occurring "when there is diminished ability to carry out important, practical social activities of daily living." While that definition is nice, it is not helpful for assessing the degree of frailty, or even its presence. It has also been described as consisting of the four primary conditions of (1) instability, (2) immobility, (3) intellectual impairment, and (4) incontinence. Today, of course, we would have to add the following condition: (5) impotence of hormones (meaning a lesser release) and male function, making five hallmark conditions related to frailty at present time.

Specialists recently came up with a working definition of frailty with more objective measures: if you have experienced weight loss, are exhausted, have weakness in grip strength, walk slowly, and have low levels of physical activity, then you likely meet the objective definition of being frail. This condition occurs in about

7 percent of all people older than fifty and, as expected, in more females than in males.

Can Frailty Be Predicted?

One of the best predictors of who is going to become frail and when is simply how well someone performs basic activities of daily living, which includes all the things you do every day. Imagine this scenario to get a better idea of what we mean: When you get up, you transfer out of bed (but you don't have to be able to walk because you can transfer from the bed to a wheelchair). You use the toilet, wash, and bathe. After dressing yourself, you sit down and eat breakfast. You then get in your car to go to work or somewhere else, and when you're halfway there, your gastrocolic reflex kicks in (likely stimulated by your breakfast), and you have to go "number two." Since your mind is working properly, you consciously control your bowels and leave nothing behind in your underpants or the car before you reach a bathroom. If you can do all these things, then you are *not* frail.

Furthermore, if you come into the hospital for any reason and these abilities are intact, you have an 82 percent chance that you likely will still be living and doing well six months later. However, if you can no longer do these simple activities, you have less than a 50 percent chance of lasting another six months, and if you actually live longer than that, you're likely to be residing in a nursing home. Performing these very simple, basic activities that we all have to do every day is a better predictor of frailty than disease. The only good other predictor is nutritional status, which is perhaps best assessed by your body mass index (BMI, discussed in Step 5). If your BMI is less than 21, meaning that you probably have lost a lot of muscle mass and strength, you likely are or will become frail. Remember that it's how skinny you are, and not how fat, that largely determines how poorly or well you do later in your life.

What Are the Causes of Frailty?

When you're young, you grow up and start to function better and better physiologically and mentally until you reach a peak around the age of twenty to twenty-five years. From then on, your functional abilities decline slowly but steadily until you reach about a hundred years. If you have a disease that is not cured or well controlled, your basic ability to function likely will go down faster. Vision, hearing, memory, sense of smell, appetite, thirst, hormones, muscle mass, and bone minerals can all be affected. These slow, physiological changes associated with getting older are the pre-frailty changes that everyone goes through to some extent from the age of fifty onward.

Frailty occurs when age-related physiological declines interact with diseases to make you less able to function in the most basic ways. It has multiple causes, including many that we have already brought to your attention, such as nutritional problems and anemia (Step 1); balance issues, declines in endurance, and muscle wasting (Step 2); weight loss (Step 5); heart failure and diabetes (Step 6); osteoporosis (Step 8); taking too many medications (Step 10); and more that are listed in the following sidebar.

Frailty is often brought on rapidly by muscular weakness. Loss of muscle mass and declining grip strength result from sarcopenia.

Potential Causes of Frailty

- Decline in overall function
- Visual problems
- Nutritional deficiencies
- Polypharmacy (taking too many medications)
- Balance problems
- Anemia (low blood levels of iron and hemoglobin)
- Congestive heart failure
- Diabetes and metabolic syndrome
- Osteoporosis (fractures)
- Sarcopenia (muscle loss)
- Decline in endurance
- Pain

About half of all people with sarcopenia are also obese, so overweight by itself will not keep you from getting frail in this case. Being overly fat with too little muscle mass to effectively move your weight around is a recipe for disaster, making the combination truly the best predictor of becoming frail early. It's hard enough to move around with a greater body weight when you have stronger, bigger muscles, but with reduced muscle mass, it can be almost impossible. Obese older women are more prone to muscular weakness, particularly if inactive.

Certain other diseases appear to speed the onset of frailty as well. For example, the metabolic syndrome, which is often the result of poor lifestyle choices such as overconsumption of calories and being sedentary, is characterized by central obesity. This type of fat within the abdomen usually leads to enhanced release of certain deleterious cytokines, such as tumor necrosis factor–alpha, from the excess fat tissue itself, the release of which can contribute to sarcopenia obesity by speeding the loss of muscle mass. These hormones are also a factor in developing this insulin resistance syndrome that leads to diabetes, hypertension, elevated blood fats, and heart disease, all of which are associated one way or another with frailty.

In reality, frailty has many more potential causes than we've discussed so far. Certainly, it results to a large extent from biological aging itself, but it's also the result of your inherent genetic makeup. Studies of centenarians have shown that some genes are protective, while others may speed up the onset of heart disease and mental declines. Since it's too late to go back and start over with new parents (to inherit a better set of genes), focus more on things within your control, such as your education level. Better-educated people generally develop frailty later or not at all, compared to less well-educated peers. This difference may be reflective of both the benefit of greater mental challenges (analogous to the mind exercises discussed in Step 4) and a greater knowledge about and likelihood of following a healthful lifestyle.

Action Steps for Better Health Tip #61

If you have experienced weight loss, are exhausted, have weakness in grip strength, walk slowly, and have low levels of physical activity, then you would likely be identified as being frail. Luckily, many of the potential causes of frailty are preventable, so learn where your risks lie and act to control these problems while you still can.

Is Frailty Preventable or Reversible?

Many of frailty's potential causes are truly preventable. For example, anorexia, lack of exercise, pain, depression, diabetes, delirium, atherosclerosis, sarcopenia, weight loss, low body weight, dehydration, heart disease, stroke, cognitive impairment, and delirium are all part of the frailty cascade, and most are treatable or preventable themselves, although the overabundance of possible causes can often make frailty difficult to completely reverse. Knowing where your risks lie and doing everything in your power to treat or control these problems early on will reduce your chances of experiencing a frail state at any point in your life.

For the best possible outcome, you should maintain your food intake, as it's still better to be a little heavy when you are older than to be too skinny. Muscle mass is heavier, and you definitely want to retain as much of it as possible for greater strength and increased mobility. As far as frailty prevention goes, doing resistance exercise is absolutely crucial and likely the most important thing you can do for your muscles, along with balance exercises. You should also try to prevent the buildup of plaque in arteries leading to the heart (and brain) with proper diet, exercise, and cholesterol-lowering medications. You should learn to recognize symptoms of depression and seek treatment early, along with treatment for chronic pain that can also stop you from being normally active. Finally, men, and possibly women, may also want to consider testosterone replacement therapies if their levels are low.

Depression Is a Reversible Cause of Frailty. Depression itself can cause symptoms of frailty, but can often be reversed. Dr. John's favorite example is the story of a furry companion of an eighty-four-year-old who died. After this individual's death, the companion became very upset, started scratching children, stopped eating, became very malnourished, and started becoming incontinent all over the house. Being worried about these behaviors, the family of the deceased companion called the veterinarian, who diagnosed the problem as senile dementia and recommended euthanasia the following day. Fortunately for this furry patient, the veterinarian talked to his wife when he went home that night. She had no medical background at all, but she suggested another possible diagnosis. She came out to the companion's house the next day, handheld the patient's paws, talked to it gently, and hand-fed it. Three months later, after excellent psychotherapy for depression, the companion had become one big, fat cat. The point of this story is that depression is perhaps a major cause of reversible symptoms of frailty, yet it is often not diagnosed by physicians (or veterinarians either, for that matter).

Action Steps for Better Health Tip #62

Some easily reversible causes of frailty include depression, cataracts, taking too many medications, anemia, low levels of certain hormones, inadequate food intake, and dehydration. Check into how to prevent or solve any of these potential causes *before* they ever become a problem.

Removing Cataracts Can Help. The development of cataracts is another example of an easily reversible cause. If you were to examine Monet's multiple paintings of the bridge across Giverny, you would see that early in his life, he painted the bridge very clearly. The bridge virtually disappeared as he became older, however, because he developed cataracts that clouded his vision. Imagine having similar visual losses and trying to find your food in the kitchen to prepare your own meals. There is almost no hope, and left to your own devices, you're likely to become malnourished. Simple things like cataracts, if they are not surgically corrected, can lead to an increased risk of frailty.

Polypharmacy Can Lead to Frailty. Even taking too many prescribed medications (called *polypharmacy* and discussed in Step 10) is a reversible cause of frailty. Vincent van Gogh always painted his physician, Dr. Gachet, with a foxglove in his hand because van Gogh had epilepsy treated with digitalis leaves prescribed by his doctor. Some of van Gogh's greatness as a painter actually resulted from being in an altered state due to the toxic nature of his drug therapy. His famous painting *Starry Night* reflects the vision of someone with classical digoxin toxicity. Too commonly, if you're older, taking digoxin, and seeing starry skies like van Gogh, your physician will likely just tell you that you're hallucinating. Eventually you will become frail from overtreatment. Keep that from happening by following the advice given in Step 10.

Boost Your Iron. It appears that anemia, defined as a hemoglobin level below 12 milligrams per deciliter (mg/dL) for women and 14 mg/dL for men, is strongly associated with frailty, dizziness with standing, falls, mental declines, and depression. Accordingly, many physicians are now treating anemic people with rEPO (a recombinant form of your body's natural hormone, erythropoietin, which boosts red blood cells) or darbepoetin (which also stimulates bone marrow to make more of these iron–containing cells) to reverse anemia and its associated frailty, with some success. If nothing else, the boost in your iron levels and red blood cells should help you feel less tired.

Charge Your Hormones. Natural reductions in hormones such as testosterone, estrogen, vitamin D, growth hormone, and DHEA over time can contribute to symptoms of frailty. Declining testosterone levels in aging males (as discussed in Step 3) are very good predictors of muscle mass losses and declines in grip strength. Clearly, testosterone replacement in aging men can play a role, but so can other hormones (e.g., vitamin D), physical activity, increased energy intake, and adequate intake of other vitamins and minerals (e.g., vitamin E) and enough fluids to prevent dehydration, all of which are easily modifiable contributing factors.

The Future of Frailty Prevention

The future of frailty prevention may include stem cell transplants to reverse sarcopenia, along with treatments that will lower levels of deleterious cytokines. Likewise, although it doesn't increase growth hormone release when taken as a supplement, ghrelin may enhance food intake and prevent declines in your ability to function well, physically and mentally, due to poor or inadequate nutrition. The fact that this hormone may also enhance memory makes it potentially one of the most exciting future treatments of age-related anorexia. Stay tuned for more exciting developments in frailty prevention in the near future.

Increase Your Daily SPA Time

"If it weren't for the fact that the TV set and the refrigerator are so far apart, some of us would get no exercise at all."
—Joey Lauren Adams, actress (1968–)

While we extolled the virtues of five types of exercise in Step 2, we must backpedal a bit now and say that exercising most days for just a short time, albeit important, is in many ways less critical than what you do during the rest of the day. To be truly effective, a formal exercise program lasting thirty minutes a day needs to be combined with more daily spontaneous physical activity (SPA), or the activities of daily living. Remember that the most critical marker of not being frail is the ability to do such activities independently, and the more active you remain, the less likely you are to lose that capacity. By way of example, in a recent study of older adults (ages seventy to eighty-two), for every 287 calories per day they expended doing anything active, they increased their chances of living longer by 68 percent. This even included doing seventy-five minutes a day of volunteering, walking at a pace of two and a half miles per hour, providing child or adult care, or doing household chores. Even if you have a while before you'll reach the age of the individuals in this study, you'll be more likely to remain looking, acting, and feeling more youthful long into your later years if you get more active yourself.

Action Steps for Better Health Tip #63

Increasing your SPA (spontaneous physical activity) will bestow innumerable health benefits, including preventing the onset of frailty. To be truly effective, a formal exercise program lasting thirty minutes a day should be combined with more daily SPA, including all activities of daily living and fidgeting.

Despite the importance of being more active in all aspects of living, most people naturally try to do as little as possible. How many times have you gone to a store and then circled around the parking lot or waited for as long as it takes to find a spot close to the door rather than just parking farther away and walking? Just recently, Dr. John saw a person get into a car near a store at one end of a parking lot and drive a distance of only fifty yards to another store on the lot's other side. Likewise, most people will wait to get on an elevator or escalator rather than make the effort to walk up or down even a single flight of stairs.

Perhaps the most sobering thought is that the universal American sport—television watching—uses almost less energy than sleeping. A study of Pima Indians, who are some of the most overweight individuals in the United States, showed that individuals that fidget frequently are less likely to gain excess fat weight than others with less spontaneous movement while sitting. It's therefore likely that everyone would benefit from adopting a "fidgeting" lifestyle.

Strategies to Increase SPA in Your Daily Life

- Park your car at the farthest point from where you are going.
- Always take the stairs; start with going down first, if necessary.
- When sitting, consciously move your legs and hands—that is, fidget more.
- Get up and move around after every thirty minutes of a sedentary activity.
- When you let your pet outside, go with it.
- Get a pedometer, and try to increase your total number of steps each day.
- Walk somewhere for fun every day.
- Consider taking public transportation whenever possible—to walk more.
- Go dancing once a week.
- Work in your garden or yard.
- Play with your children or grandchildren.
- Think of other creative ways to move more throughout the day.

A peptide called orexin in the hypothalamus, which is the part of the brain that controls food intake and thirst, was recently discovered. What makes it important is that it apparently increases spontaneous activity in rodents. Ever since its discovery, the pharmaceutical industry has been searching for a similar compound that people could simply swallow in drug form to enhance their SPA to keep from gaining fat weight. Both of us, though, wonder why we all can't simply consciously increase our daily movement, a choice with only positive side effects on overall health. If you make it a priority to increase your SPA, it's possible that at some point you'll continue doing so without giving it a thought.

The reality, unfortunately, is that a high level of conscious thought about SPA may be needed for an extended time to truly change human behavior. For example, in one study, researchers noted that at a local Philadelphia-area mall, everyone took the escalators instead of the stairs located next to them. To try to increase SPA, the investigators posted a sign with a picture of a heart running up the stairs to remind people of the health benefits of stair climbing. In response, large numbers of shoppers started taking the stairs—at least until a week after the sign was taken down. Without a constant reminder to be more active, almost all of the shoppers reverted back to standing on the escalators and being transported with minimal effort on their part.

What can you do to easily increase your daily activity? Try following some or all of the suggestions found in the sidebar "Strategies to Increase SPA in Your Daily Life," on the previous page, to get more active.

A Final Word About Step 9

Many falls can be prevented if you do balance exercises, increase the strength of your lateral quadriceps muscles, and correct your visual defects. In addition, if you fall frequently, consider using hip pads to reduce your risk of bone fractures. Falling can be a symptom of frailty, a complex condition that results in a decreased ability to function well enough to do normal activities of daily living. Recognize the reversible causes of this condition, such as depression, anemia, anorexia, and physical inactivity, and treat them as early as possible to stay healthy and strong for longer. Finally, get more active on a daily basis by doing more spontaneous activities to enhance and maintain your overall health, vitality, and youthful vigor.

10

Keep an Eye on Prevention

"Prevention is better than cure."
—*Charles Dickens (1812–1870) in* Martin Chuzzlewit

As we touched on in the previous step, one of the keys to feeling younger and more vital for longer is to prevent health problems like frailty before they ever happen to you. You really need to know where you currently stand and which direction to head in to stay in optimal health, both physically and mentally. In addition to giving you some tools to assess your current health and determine which preventive measures you may need to take, this final step also teaches you how to assess the safety of your medications and gives you guidelines to follow on your journey to greater longevity, increased energy levels, a higher quality of living, and better overall health for as long as you live.

Improving Your Biological Age

Maybe you really can tap into a fountain of youth so you can live as long and as well as you possibly can. If so, the chances are that the fountain contains different cures due to each person's uniqueness. The good news is that regardless of whether or not your journey has already brought you to this elixir of eternal life (we're guessing probably not), you can still make a big difference in how youthful you remain from here on out.

No matter what your current chronological age is, you can take steps to improve your biological status, even if your lifestyle isn't perfect. For instance, having diabetes that is not effectively controlled accelerates aging, resulting in an average loss of twelve years of life and a decrease in quality of life for twenty of those remaining years. On the other hand, controlling your blood sugar levels effectively in a normal or near normal range can prevent almost all of these potential, negative consequences.

Action Steps for Better Health Tip #64

You can do many things to lower your biological age, including becoming more educated, earning more money, coping positively with stress, being in a committed relationship, seeking out spirituality, controlling chronic diseases, and not smoking. Start improving your health now by taking small steps in the right direction.

Effectively controlling diabetes is just one example of how you can dramatically influence the effect that chronic diseases have on your biological age, but there are many others. Simply stopping smoking greatly lowers your risk of heart disease, lung cancer, and many more age-enhancing chronic problems. Preventing constipation may even help by reducing the risk of colon cancer. What's more, many other chronic conditions that can make you feel older than you are may be improved or even prevented by changes in lifestyle, even in middle age or later (see Table 10.1).

Not all positive interventions are related to your physical health. In fact, your mental status is largely affected by your outlook on life and how you handle stress and other hurdles that life hands you. Your biological age is actually improved by having a higher level of education, earning more money in your job (but probably only up to a point), being in a committed relationship (e.g., mar-

TABLE 10.1 Strategies to Prevent or Control
Age-Accelerating Conditions

Disease or Condition	Prevention Strategies
Heart disease and stroke	Control high blood pressure. Quit smoking. Lose excess fat weight before age 60. Reduce intake of saturated and trans fats and cholesterol. Increase intake of fish. Exercise more. Consider having 1–2 alcoholic drinks daily.
Cancer	Quit smoking. Reduce intake of dietary fat and salt- or smoke-cured meats. Minimize sun and radiation exposure. Increase fiber in diet. Exercise regularly.
Emphysema and chronic bronchitis	Quit smoking, and avoid exposure to secondhand smoke.
Diabetes mellitus	Control blood glucose levels. Follow a diet high in fiber and unsaturated fats. Improve the overall quality of diet. Exercise regularly. Lose 5–7 percent of body weight, but only if exercising at the same time.
Gallstones	Lose excess fat weight.
High blood pressure	Lose excess fat weight. Use no extra salt, and restrict intake of salty foods. Exercise regularly. Quit smoking. Maintain adequate calcium and magnesium intake.
Osteoarthritis	Exercise regularly, including moderate resistance exercises. Lose excess body fat if under 60, but retain muscle mass.
Osteoporosis	Maintain adequate calcium and vitamin D intake. Exercise regularly. Drink alcohol no more than moderately. Watch intake of animal proteins, salt, colas, and caffeine.
Constipation	Drink adequate fluids (4–6 glasses a day). Increase fiber intake. Exercise regularly. Use the bathroom following meals, when you're helped by reflexes.

ried people live longer), and seeking out your spiritual side, either through religious involvement or other avenues.

Taking Control of Your Own Preventive Health

Your health is likely to suffer unless you take responsibility for it yourself. A large part of being in charge of your personal health is having the knowledge to ask the right questions when you visit your doctor. As mentioned in earlier discussions, certain biomark-

Questions to Ask for the Best Preventive Health Care

- Is your blood pressure in a normal range, or should it be lower?
- Is your fasting blood glucose below 100 mg/dL, and is it higher than at your last checkup (i.e., trending upward)?
- What is your total cholesterol, and how high are your levels of HDL and LDL (sd LDL in particular)?
- Are your thyroid hormone levels normal, especially that of your thyroid stimulating hormone (TSH)?
- Has your weight changed since your last visit?
- Are you getting shorter compared to your height at twenty years of age?
- Would a screening test for osteoporosis be appropriate?
- Are your medications still working well for you, and is it possible to take fewer, especially if you're taking more than five regularly?
- Are your vaccinations up-to-date? (You should consider a flu shot every year, pneumococcal every six years, tetanus once a decade, and herpes zoster once.)
- Is it time to have your stool tested or retested for blood?
- Given your history, are any other screening tests (for cancer or anything else) warranted for you?

ers of aging let you know what areas to work on. The sidebar "Questions to Ask for the Best Preventive Health Care" provides you with a list of questions that would be helpful for the best prevention and identification of treatable health problems.

Early Screening Can Improve and Extend Your Life

Each of us has a great deal of control over our own health, so don't let anyone tell you otherwise. Traditionally, doctors have viewed good health as simply the absence of disease. As you live longer, it really needs a broader definition. Think of your health during the rest of your life as being affected by three related factors: (1) absence of disease; (2) maintenance of optimal function—that is, a younger biological age; and (3) an adequate support system. Defining good health in this manner places more emphasis on your quality of life: feeling good enough to be able to do the things that you want to. This is exactly where we think it should be. Even if you develop a chronic health condition at some point, you can still lead an enjoyable and productive life with the second and third factors in mind.

Screening and monitoring are important keys to maintaining an optimal quality of life and improved health. Continuing a combination of screening to find problems early enough and monitoring your progress in their treatment can alert your doctor to a health issue before it has a chance to become serious and potentially less treatable. If either a screening test or new symptoms raise any questions about your health, further testing can be done to determine the extent of the problem and the best course of action. Once you have a diagnosed health problem, regular follow-up becomes a vital part of keeping it from worsening and taking away from your quality of life or your longevity.

Doctors recommend screening for treatable conditions that can significantly impact your health, particularly when they are asymptomatic and more easily corrected if you find them early. An example of a good screening test is a colonoscopy to detect small polyps or early cancerous tumors in your large intestine that would otherwise be undetectable until the cancer became more advanced.

Action Steps for Better Health Tip #65

To make your good health last, screen for treatable conditions that can be cured upon early detection. Even if you develop a chronic health condition, you can still lead an enjoyable and productive life as long as you control it and keep your body running well, and particularly if you have a good support system, such as a caring spouse.

How often you should be screened depends on you—your genetic makeup, family history, personal habits, and lifestyle. It would be ideal to be screened for all possible diseases, but doing so would be highly impractical, time-consuming, and costly. If you have a greater risk for developing certain conditions (e.g., your family may have a strong history of colorectal cancer), screening for these potential problems would be sensible. You may decide it's not worthwhile to check for others that you have little risk for, at least not on a regular basis. Ultimately, it is up to you and your doctor to determine which are your highest risk conditions and how often you should be screened.

What Medications Can and Can't Do for Your Health

According to some individuals, a man's health can be judged by what he takes two at a time, pills or steps! Certainly, a healthy lifestyle by itself can reduce your dependency on pills, but there is a place for many medications in the effective management of chronic health problems. They can be naturally occurring or man-made and include not only prescribed medications but also caffeine, alcohol, nicotine, and over-the-counter pain relievers, along with a variety of illicit substances, such as marijuana and cocaine, and unproven herbal products like saw palmetto and Saint John's wort. In short, drugs are not just what the doctor prescribes for you.

Action Steps for Better Health Tip #66

Medications include not only prescribed ones but also caffeine, alcohol, nicotine, drugstore pain relievers, recreational drugs, and herbal products. A number of these substances may cause untoward side effects from drug interactions or allergies. Staying on top of your medications and any symptoms they cause is critical to maintaining good health, particularly if you take two or more medications daily.

Keep in mind that there is no such thing as an absolutely safe drug, even if you take only "natural" ones. Every one of them, whether an over-the-counter cough syrup or an established antibiotic, can produce side effects—some of them undesirable—when taken with certain other medications or foods or if the body has an allergic reaction to the substance. Staying on top of your medications and any symptoms they cause is critical to your lasting health and staying young.

Some safety precautions related to medication use are listed in the sidebar "Keeping Your Medication Use Safe and Effective."

Keeping Your Medication Use Safe and Effective

DO List

- DO follow instructions on container labels.
- DO have container labels with print that is large enough to read easily.
- DO have a list of all the drugs you take, including over-the-counter drugs, herbal remedies, and vitamins, and provide it to your health care providers at each visit.
- DO keep all the times and doses straight, and carry a list of your medications, the doses, and why you take them with you at all times.
- DO include all drug allergies you have experienced on your medication list.
- DO wear some type of medical alert jewelry for important drugs, like insulin or antiepilepsy medications.

DON'T List

- DON'T transfer medications to unmarked containers or containers labeled with directions for other drugs.
- DON'T take drugs without reading the labels first.
- DON'T use out-of-date medicines or reuse old prescriptions.
- DON'T share your medicines with anyone else or take someone else's prescription.

Although using only the original prescription containers is a safe practice, it may also be wise to use a weekly pill sorter, the type that has an individual container for each day of the week. By putting your week's worth of medications into the appropriate daily slots, it will be easier to keep track of whether or not you have taken your medications on any given day. If you take them more than once a day, having separate pill sorters for morning and evening doses would also be advantageous.

Could Taking Too Many Medications Actually Be Harming You?

You may be experiencing polypharmacy if you're taking more than five medications daily. Taking too many different drugs for your various health conditions (e.g., high cholesterol, diabetes, elevated systolic blood pressure, postmenopausal symptoms) can lead to a vicious cycle of taking multiple drugs to address the same problem or to counteract symptoms caused by their interactions. Thus, the "cure" may be causing some of the problem. If you ever find yourself in this situation, have your doctor review what you're currently taking, including any over-the-counter medicines, vitamins, and herbal supplements (all of which can also alter the effects of prescription drugs), to reduce the potential for side effects or harmful interactions. If it's possible to cut back, you should, but don't refuse to take a medication that you really need. It may also be possible to try using an alternate medication to treat a specific health issue.

Action Steps for Better Health Tip #67

If you're taking too many medications, which is usually more than five a day, the cure may be worse than the problem. Side effects from drug interactions can occur, even if you take as few as two medications a day. Talk to your doctor about cutting back on the number of daily drugs in such cases.

Risk Factors for Adverse Drug Reactions and Interactions

- **Age:** The older you are, the greater your chance for a drug reaction.
- **Genes:** Having certain genetic traits may make you more likely to experience an adverse reaction.
- **Number of daily medications:** The more drugs you take, the greater your chances of suffering side effects and potentially adverse drug interactions, particularly if you take more than five drugs a day.
- **Drug dosage:** Almost four-fifths of all drug reactions are dose related.
- **History of adverse reactions:** If you have had an adverse drug reaction in the past, even when taking a different drug, your risk is greater.
- **Hospitals:** Medication mistakes are common in hospitals, so when you are given a drug to take, make sure it was specifically prescribed for you.

The risk factors for adverse drug reactions given in the sidebar emphasize the importance of informing your doctor about all your medications and any allergies or previous drug reactions you've had. Also, always ask about new medications and why each is being prescribed. If you have more than one doctor, give a complete list of your medications—or bring the medications themselves—to each doctor.

As you get older, your liver and kidneys may not process drugs as effectively, and you may retain them in your body longer. The result is that taking a dose that is safe for a twenty-year-old may be too much for you at fifty or sixty years of age. Consequently, it's possible to have drug interactions, even if you're only taking two medications. In addition, when you have select preexisting health problems, taking certain medications, which may be for other conditions, can actually make your health worse. Take the following precautions to heart:

- If you have chronic constipation, avoid the use of calcium channel antagonists, imipramine, amitriptyline, and doxepin (the latter three are antidepressants).
- If you have seizures, don't take Wellbutrin (an antidepressant).
- If you are hypertensive, avoid medications containing pseudoephedrine, which is found in many over-the-counter decongestant drugs such as Sudafed.
- If you have peptic ulcer disease, avoid aspirin and other nonsteroidal anti-inflammatory drugs, such as ibuprofen (Nuprin, Advil).
- If you suffer from Parkinson's disease, you should avoid Reglan and many antipsychotic drugs.
- If you have low levels of sodium in your blood, known as hyponatremia, you should not be taking Paxil, Zoloft, Luvox, or Celexa.

How medications work in your body can also change over time. The sidebar on the following page provides a list of drugs best avoided by older individuals.

Some medications should be taken with food or after meals to decrease the chance of stomach irritation, while others should be taken on an empty stomach (meaning at least one hour before eating or two hours after eating). Also, don't be afraid to discuss cost openly with your doctor. If a medication is too expensive, say so rather than just "forgetting" to get it from the drugstore. There may be alternatives, including other brands or generic equivalents, which are less expensive. Newer drugs being pushed on your doctors by pharmaceutical company reps are not necessarily more effective than cheaper, older drugs either. Inquire about possible alternatives.

Beers List of Drugs to Be Avoided as You Get Older

- amiodarone (Cordarone, except during short hospitalizations)
- amitriptyline (Elavil, Endep)
- antianxiety drugs (Xanax, Valium, and Librium)
- antipsychotics, unless schizophrenic or having paranoia, illusions, delusions, or hallucinations
- barbiturates (except phenobarbital, brand name Solfoton)
- Bisacodyl and Cascara (laxatives, not for long-term use)
- chlorpropamide (Diabinese)
- chlorpheniramine (Chlor-Trimeton)
- cyproheptadine (Periactin)
- desiccated thyroid
- diphenhydramine hydrochloride (Benadryl, found in over-the-counter drugs)
- disopyramide (Norpace)
- docusate (Colace, Correctol, Ex-Lax, and Peri-Colace)
- doxazosin (Cardura)
- estrogens, in women over sixty years old
- fluoxetine daily (Prozac)
- imipramine (Tofranil)
- meperidine (Demerol)
- methyldopa (Aldomet)
- methyltestosterone (Android-10, Testred, Virilon)
- nifedipine short-acting (Procardia, Adalat)
- propoxyphene (Darvon, Darvocet)

Source: Fick, D. M., Cooper, J. W., Wade, W. E., Waller, J. L., Maclean, J. R., and Beers, M. H. (2003). Updating the Beers criteria for potentially inappropriate medication use in older adults: Results of a US consensus panel of experts. *Arch Intern Med*, 163(22), 2716–24.

How Easy Is It to Take Too Many Drugs?

A number of beliefs about the ability of medications to cure everything that ails you may contribute to polypharmacy. The ones that follow can significantly impact your choice to take more drugs, but usually not in a good way.

Belief #1: If one dose makes me feel good, a larger dose will make me feel better. Always discuss dose changes with your doctor, and don't alter them yourself. Even small increases in your doses can cause unwanted or dangerous side effects.

Belief #2: If a drug doesn't help, I need to add another one. Every time another drug is added, it increases your chance of having a drug reaction. Taking nonprescription medications—even cold medicines or decongestants—without telling your doctor also raises the likelihood of an adverse interaction.

Belief #3: If I can get a medication without a prescription, it must be safe. Nonprescription drugs are still drugs. For example, drugstore decongestants can worsen bladder problems associated with an enlarged prostate gland, antacids can interfere with drug and vitamin absorption, and aspirin can prevent normal blood clotting. If you're taking iron for the treatment of anemia, ingesting it at the same time as your calcium supplements may block the iron's absorption. Moreover, even natural or herbal preparations like Saint-John's wort, an herbal remedy for mild depression, can interact with prescription medications for depression.

Belief #4: If I have used this medicine for years, I must need it now. The effects of a drug you have taken daily for many years, such as a blood pressure medication, won't alter significantly in one day but can over a longer time frame. If you begin taking a new drug, the effectiveness of the first drug or how you respond to it may also change. Some alterations in your body's response to drugs can be anticipated as part of the normal process of getting older, but others may be caused by diseases of the heart, liver, or kidneys. Also, be cautious when taking medications you use only occasionally, such as antihistamines, sleeping pills, or pain relievers, because as you grow older your body may react differently to them.

Belief #5: If it helped someone else, it can help me, too. Never borrow medicine from friends or relatives to see if it works for you. Taking another person's medicines can be dangerous. By way of example, suppose you notice that your feet tend to swell by the end of the day, so you borrow a drug from a friend whose feet have the same problem, but due to a heart condition. If your swelling is the result of something else, your friend's drug probably won't help you, and it may even cause dangerous side effects such as low blood pressure or fainting.

Action Steps for Better Health Tip #68

Geriatricians are doctors who specialize in health care related to aging, and they may be better than family physicians at providing special care for older individuals and for giving advice on how to prevent future problems. Plan on seeing one if you're between sixty-five and seventy years of age and symptomatic.

When Should You See a Geriatrician?

For day-to-day problems and major medical illnesses, your family practitioner or internist is the appropriate doctor to visit, along with a specialist if you need to. Geriatricians, however, are better at providing special care when older individuals are having chronic health problems, and they can also give excellent advice on preventive aging. By the time you are between sixty-five and seventy years of age, you would probably benefit from seeing a geriatric specialist for a comprehensive assessment to see if you have any potential or existing problems that are treatable. But be prepared to spend one to three hours at the visit. Consult the sidebar "When Should You Visit a Geriatrician?" to help you decide when the time is right.

When Should You Visit a Geriatrician?

If you are older than seventy years of age, see a geriatrician if you

- Take nine or more medications daily
- Are fatigued frequently or all the time
- Are having memory problems
- Are having falls for unexplained reasons
- Are feeling sad
- Can no longer do your activities of daily living (e.g., showering, fixing meals)
- Are unhappy with the answers you are getting from your regular physician
- Score positively on the ADAM questionnaire given in Step 3 (men only)

A Final Word About Step 10

To ensure your optimal health and longer-lasting feelings of youthfulness, you need to stay current on new treatment options and preventive medicine. Screening for early detection and prevention of certain medical conditions is also a key to living well for longer and maintaining better health. Preventing and treating such conditions early can prevent you from feeling biologically older. Be informed about all of your medical conditions, ask your doctor questions, and be alert for any symptoms that may develop from your health problems or the use of medications. If you're taking five or more medications, talk to your doctor about reducing the number to prevent possible problems from drug interactions. Finally, schedule a checkup in the near future to stay on top of your health while you have the chance to have the greatest positive impact.

Conclusion

A Glimpse into the Future

"The greatest business of life is to be, to do, to do without, and to depart."

—*John Morley, British statesman (1838–1923)*

As we have said from the beginning, your journey through life involves many possible alternate paths for looking and feeling your best for longer. We hope that the information provided in this book will make your decisions easier. Although we laid out the known paths, it's harder to describe for you possible alternate choices that may become readily available in the not-so-distant future. In concluding, however, we will provide you with a glimpse of some of the possibilities looming on the horizon that may serve to enhance your health and longevity.

Claims About Antiaging Medicine

For many years, the search for the mythical fountain of youth has led to unscrupulous people selling their version of snake oil to vulnerable individuals desperate to slow the inevitable signs of getting older, and modern times are no exception. Just recently, pseudoscientific claims associated with growth hormone and dehydroepiandrosterone (DHEA, discussed in Step 3) as agents that will "reverse the aging process" have regularly been appearing in countless newspapers, magazines, and books.

Many of these antiaging claims are based on flawed research studies, while others stem from published but unproven hypotheses by scientists that were later touted as fact by the lay press. For example, the claim by scientist Linus Pauling that megadoses of vitamin C will protect cells from free-radical damage remains alive today in spite of mounting evidence suggesting that instead of prolonging life, supplemental megadoses of most vitamins—including his beloved vitamin C—may instead shorten it. On the other hand, stem cells are a promising therapy that might reverse the signs of aging in muscles and cure Alzheimer's disease.

The Future of Getting the Right Drug

Pharmacogenomics is a fledgling field of study focused on finding out what influence your unique genetic makeup may have on how well a certain drug works for you and whether you're likely to experience side effects. For example, someday your doctor may be able to tell from your genetic makeup whether statins used to lower blood cholesterol will work for you, or if an alternate drug would be better to resolve your health problems. Due to genetic differences, your liver may be able to get rid of drugs more quickly than someone else's, thereby lowering the risk of harmful side effects. Once this science advances far enough to allow for better testing of these gene differences, physicians will then be able to vary the prescription of drugs as necessary to match the unique characteristics of each person and medical condition.

Environmental Interactions with Your Genome

The environment can also modulate gene expression. For starters, we know that head injury accelerates Alzheimer's disease in people with certain genes. These genes are the same ones that increase risk for heart disease, particularly in smokers. Similarly, the interaction of a major life stressor with other genetic traits may increase the likelihood that someone will experience major depression.

Even physical activity produces different responses depending on the person's genotype, with some individuals responding more than others.

These simple examples represent only the beginning of the exploration of gene and environment interactions, both of which play a role in determining whether you will stay biologically younger than someone else your age. The new social science of aging in the twenty-first century will require the inclusion of a person's genetic background to allow full interpretation of potential environmental effects.

Aging Rates in Mice, Men, and Flies

Until now, researchers have studied genes that underlie aging in a single animal, such as flies or mice, or in different human tissues without finding the answers to enigmas such as why tortoises and rockfish are still young at an age when humans are not. A protein associated with aging in one species may not be relevant in a different animal, which makes it difficult to find aging processes that are universal across species. At the other end of the spectrum, flies die off before humans can go through infancy, making it clear that not all cells reach their reproductive limit at the same rate. And why do flies' cells self-destruct in a matter of weeks if tortoises can live hundreds of years?

Researchers at the Stanford University School of Medicine have found something at the core of this cellular aging process: a group of genes that are consistently less active in older animals across a variety of species. Moreover, their activity is a consistent indicator of how far a cell has progressed toward its eventual end. These recent findings overturn the commonly held view that all animals, including humans, age like an abandoned property— slowly but surely deteriorating over time and without a master plan for the decay. It now appears that there is indeed a master design built into your cells determining how long they will live and prosper.

Genes that are more active are thought to be making more proteins. According to these findings, a cell keeps up repairs until a predetermined time, after which decay happens as a matter of course. In tortoise cells, these repairs may be kept up for hundreds of years, delaying the decay. Fly cells, however, reach this process within weeks. Although we still don't know what exactly triggers that process, we now have a way of detecting the point a cell has reached in its life span limit. These researchers looked at which genes were actively producing protein and at what level, examining flies, mice, and tissues taken from the muscle, brain, and kidney of eighty-one adults of all ages. Interestingly, one group of genes consistently made less protein as cells aged in all of the animals and tissues. These genes make up the cellular machinery called the electron transport chain, which generates energy in the cell's powerhouses, the mitochondria.

This gene activity is a better indicator of a cell's relative biological age than anything else found to date. For instance, one forty-one-year-old participant had gene activity similar to that of people ten to twenty years older; also, muscle tissue from the same person was similarly prematurely aged. Conversely, the sample from a sixty-four-year-old, whose muscles looked like those of a person thirty years younger, also showed gene activity patterns similar to a younger person. These results confirm prior assumptions that the rate of aging is at least in part genetically determined. Participants whose tissues appeared younger than their true age had something special—and dearly sought by aging researchers—that made their cells continue to activate genes in a more youthful pattern.

What causes the electron transport chain genes to slow their protein production, and why does it happen? Is there anything we can do to reverse or prevent this process in humans? The main researcher of this study suggested that aging wouldn't have to happen if cells weren't programmed to fail. Using specific markers for biological aging, he thinks future research will reveal what drives the process and possibly how to alter its course. While death and taxes have been unavoidable, in the case of aging, someday the former may no longer be true.

Become an Advocate for Helping People Age Gracefully

"The test of a people is how it behaves toward the old. It is easy to love children. Even tyrants and dictators make a point of being fond of children. But affection and care for the old, the uncurable, the helpless are the true gold mines of a culture."

—*Rabbi Abraham Joshua Heschel (1907–1972) in* The Insecurity of Freedom

In 2006, the year that both Bill Clinton and Dr. John, together with the first wave of baby boomers, reached their sixtieth year and took the first tentative steps toward their golden years, Dr. John observed all around him the ugly specter of ageism. Congress unfunded the Geriatric Education Centers and cut the reimbursement for Medicare Part D. In academic medical centers, he saw little movement toward increasing teaching about how to age successfully and stay feeling good for longer. Instead, professors were choosing to focus on esoteric high technology and new drugs of uncertain benefit.

While everywhere angels were singing about the need to concentrate on the future care of our older population, Dr. John failed to see a harkening of the public to the message. Even his peers appeared more inclined to look toward maintaining their immortality rather than toward setting up the means to allow themselves to maintain a younger biological age into their twilight years. While none of us can conclude our autobiography until we die, it currently appears that we're writing one where disaster awaits us at the end of our journey of life.

What needs to be done to improve the situation? In the United States, the flow of the mighty dollar often appears to be the only way to bring about change. We recommend that in 2008 and beyond, Congress give up its ageist attitudes and pass legislation to increase the Medicare rate by 20 percent, give medical schools funds to allow geriatricians increased time for teaching, re-fund the Geriatric Education Centers at twice their previous level, increase funding for the National Institute on Aging, and move rapidly toward a universal computerized medical record.

You may legitimately ask Dr. John what he's been smoking, or if he has just developed early signs of mild cognitive impairment! Nevertheless, he strongly believes that it is time for America's baby boomer population to begin to advocate its own better future, simply by inundating Congress with letters, e-mails, and phone calls (contact information can be found at senate.gov and at house .gov). Only in this way will our remaining years be better for us than it was for those who went through it before us. As Rabbi Abraham Joshua Heschel also said, "Man lives in a spiritual order. Moments of insight, moments of decision, moments of prayer may be insignificant in the world of space, yet they put life into focus." It is time for decision and prayer, coupled with action, to reverse the tendencies to treat the older generations with less respect and honor than they deserve, which is what we are currently experiencing in our society.

A Warning About the Quest for Immortality

You've all heard the saying, "Be careful what you wish for." The problem with wishing for, and getting, eternal life is illustrated by a Greek myth about Tithonus, a handsome but mortal youth who was also the morning lover of Aurora, the goddess of dawn. Realizing that she would live forever, Aurora prevailed on her father Zeus to grant Tithonus immortality, but forgot to ask for his eternal youth as well. To her great mortification, as time went on she began to discern that her lover was growing old. When Tithonus reached fifty, his libido was a problem; at seventy, his potency declined; by eighty, he shuffled around her castle with a stoop; and by one hundred, his memory was shot. Love's youthful bloom gone from her lover, Aurora could no longer stand him, but as he had immortality, she was stuck with him. As the myth goes, hearing him muttering incessantly one day, she flew into a rage and turned him into a grasshopper. So the next time you hear a grasshopper chirping, remember that it's just the sound of an old man babbling on and on. Immortality may not be all that it's cracked up to be!

If Your Personal Quest for Immortality Is Still Alive and Kicking

For those of you who still wish to continue your personal quest for immortality, we suggest you read the book *Fantastic Voyage* by Ray Kurzweil and Terry Grossman. This book takes a science fiction approach to radical life extension. Kurzweil, a brilliant computer expert and futurist, believes that human beings will eventually become immortal by fusing with computers—making "hubots"—and having nanobots circulating in our bloodstream to remove cancerous cells and other toxic substances. To allow himself to reach this questionably wonderful future today, he takes about 250 "nutritional" pills a day, along with a variety of intravenous therapies once a week. As he squanders his money and life on these radical, supposedly life-extending therapies, he claims that his faith in the regimen grows at an exponential pace equivalent to the growth of computing power.

From his other books, it would seem that Kurzweil's concept of intelligent design is that sometime in the twenty-first century, computerized robots will become the next great evolutionary step, and any of us who survive will become beloved pets of these superior machines! However outlandish this may sound, many of his ideas on computer interfaces with humans are already becoming reality. We already implant computers into the cochlea to enhance hearing, attempts are being made to put computer chips into the retina to allow the blind to see, and electrical stimulation allows people with severe Parkinson's disease to work. In addition, we're seeing amazing advances in the use of robotics to replace lost limbs. The future will be extraordinarily interesting, but it remains highly unpredictable.

Putting It All Together

Whether robotics or other technological advances are in your health-related future or not, congratulations are in order! Having read through this book, you now have the knowledge to help you live your life to the max, all while enjoying a more youthful body and improved health. Immortality, if you should find a way to achieve it, is irrelevant if you don't have your health. Unfortunately, you still have to put the easy steps suggested here into practice to live well, and changing lifelong habits can be a bit challenging. In anticipation of your need for a refresher from time to time, we have summarized the main points of our basic prescription for a long and happy life, as follows:

- Eat fish at least four times a week, and if you have elevated cholesterol or heart disease, also consider taking fish oil supplements daily.
- Drink no more than one to two glasses of red wine or other alcoholic beveraages each day.
- Eat adequate amounts of protein and calories, along with plenty of tea, fiber, and antioxidant-rich foods such as whole grains, leafy vegetables, legumes, spices, and dark chocolate.
- Exercise for thirty minutes daily, making sure that you do all five kinds of exercise (endurance, resistance, balance, flexibility, and posture) each week.
- Take 1,000 to 1,200 milligrams of calcium and 800 international units of vitamin D from age fifty onward if female, age sixty-five onward if male, and have your bone mineral density and vitamin D levels measured regularly.
- For women having hot flashes, take low-dose estradiol (estrogen supplement) and a natural progestin for five years,

and if you have your ovaries removed, take just the estrogen until you reach age fifty-five.

- For men, check your ADAM score (Step 3), and if it's positive, get screened for depression, have your bioavailable testosterone level measured, and consider taking testosterone supplements if it's low.

- If you're having memory problems, consider taking 600 milligrams of alpha-lipoic acid daily, but also do frequent memory exercises to sharpen your mind.

- Keep active and happy, maintain a positive spiritual life, and if you enjoy organized religion, go to church regularly—rather than watching televangelists from home.

- Aim to keep your weight stable, since neither large amounts of weight gain nor of weight loss is good for you as you age.

- Make sure your physician measures your good-bad cholesterol (large, fluffy LDL), and if this component explains why your total cholesterol level is high, don't have it lowered too much with medications. If your cholesterol is elevated from sd LDL, the bad-bad kind, however, then medications will help protect your vessels.

- If you're at high risk for certain types of cancer or other health problems and screening tests are available, get screened regularly to detect problems early.

- Enhance your exercise time with spontaneous physical activity (SPA) to prevent falls and frailty.

Most of all, remember that your ultimate goal is to maintain optimal health, a younger biological age, and a high quality of life for as long as you live, which shouldn't be a problem now that you have at your fingertips the most up-to-date information possible on how to do so. Question your doctor's opinion, continue to educate yourself, be your own advocate, enjoy life, and smile your way to the century mark and beyond!

Appendix

Saint Louis University Mental Status (SLUMS) Examination

Since determining what constitutes normal cognitive function as you get older and what is not can often be difficult, simple tools are needed to assist in diagnosing mild cognitive impairment (MCI) and dementia. Accordingly, researchers including Dr. John have developed a validated measure, the Saint Louis University Mental Status Examination (SLUMS), which can be used to determine a person's level of cognitive decline. It is important to remember that a person's level of education may also affect performance; thus, the scoring of the test takes into account whether an individual completed high school. Although this exam is normally used by clinicians like Dr. John, you can still have someone give you the SLUMS and score it for you to get a better idea where you stand.

Saint Louis University Mental Status (SLUMS) Examination

Name _____ Age _____

Is patient alert? _____ Level of education _____

1. What day of the week is it? ①   ___ /1
2. What is the year? ①   ___ /1
3. What state are we in? ①   ___ /1
4. Please remember these five objects. I will ask you what they are later.
   Apple   Pen   Tie   House   Car
5. You have $100, and you go to the store and buy a dozen apples for $3 and a tricycle for $20.
   How much did you spend? ①
   How much do you have left? ②   ___ /3
6. Please name as many animals as you can in one minute.
   0–4 animals ⓪   5–9 animals ①   10–14 animals ②   15+ animals ③   ___ /3
7. What were the five objects I asked you to remember? One point for each one correct.   ___ /5
8. I am going to give you a series of numbers and I would like you to give them to me backward. For example, if I say 42, you would say 24.
   ⓪ 87   ① 649   ① 8537   ___ /2
9. This is a clock face. Please put in the hour markers and the time at ten minutes to eleven o'clock.
   Hour markers OK ②
   Time correct ②   ___ /4
10. Please place an X in the triangle. ①
    Which of the above figures is largest? ①   ___ /2
11. I am going to tell you a story. Please listen carefully because afterward, I'm going to ask you some questions about it.

    Jill was a very successful stockbroker. She made a lot of money on the stock market. She then met Jack, a devastatingly handsome man. She married him and had three children. They lived in Chicago. She then stopped work and stayed at home to bring up her children. When they were teenagers, she went back to work. She and Jack lived happily ever after.

    What was the female's name? ②   What work did she do? ②
    When did she go back to work? ②   What state did she live in? ②   ___ /8

TOTAL SCORE _____

SCORING		
High School Education		**Less than High School Education**
27–30	Normal	25–30
21–26	MNCD*	20–24
1–20	Dementia	1–19

*Mild neurocognitive disorder.

Developed by Tariq, S., N. Tumosa, J. T. Chibnall, H. M. Perry III, and J. E. Morley. Used with permission.

Resources for Healthy Living

Aging Successfully
Dr. John Morley's newsletters and online information on aging.
medschool.slu.edu/agingsuccessfully
e-mail: aging@slu.edu

American Heart Association
Information on cardiovascular diseases and hypertension.
americanheart.org
americanheart.org/presenter.jhtml?identifier=3021399 (blood pressure quiz)

American Society on Aging
The largest organization of professionals in the field of aging, which has online resources, publications, and educational opportunities.
asaging.org/index.cfm

American Stroke Association
Information about strokes.
strokeassociation.org

Cancer Treatment, Prevention, and Advocacy Information
aicr.org (American Institute for Cancer Research)
americancancersociety.org or cancer.org

canceradvocacy.org
cancer.gov (National Cancer Institute)
mayoclinic.org
oncology.com (People Living with Cancer)
preventcancer.org

Center for Grief Care and Education at San Diego Hospice and Palliative Care
sdhospice.org/cgcefpc.htm

Cyberounds
An Internet-based educational program for physicians and health care providers offering regular updates on geriatrics.
cyberounds.com

The Doctor Will See You Now.com
Senior Living articles (including Dr. John's).
thedoctorwillseeyounow.com/articles/senior_living

Dr. John Morley's website
drjohnmorley.com

Dr. Sheri Colberg's website
Exercise information, particularly related to diabetes.
shericolberg.com

"Exercise: A Guide from the National Institute on Aging and the National Aeronautics and Space Administration"
weboflife.nasa.gov/exerciseandaging/cover.html

GenAge
Human aging genomic resources.
genomics.senescence.info/genes

The Longevity Consortium
Consortium of scientists sharing genetic research on aging.
longevityconsortium.org

Medline Plus
Current health information on over seven hundred topics and drugs, provided by the U.S. National Library of Medicine and the National Institutes of Health (NIH).
medlineplus.gov

Mercury Levels in Commercial Fish and Shellfish (USFDA)
cfsan.fda.gov/~frf/sea-mehg.html

National Cholesterol Education Program
Heart attack risk calculator.
hp2010.nhlbihin.net/atpiii/calculator.asp

National Osteoporosis Foundation
nof.org

Real Age.com
Includes the "Real Age Test" to estimate biological age.
realage.com

Recommended Reading

Beare, Sally. *50 Secrets of the World's Longest Living People*. New York, NY: Marlowe and Company, 2006.

Becker, Gretchen. *The First Year Type 2 Diabetes: An Essential Guide for the Newly Diagnosed*. 2nd ed. New York: Marlowe and Company, 2007.

Colberg, Sheri R., and Steven V. Edelman. *50 Secrets of the Longest Living People with Diabetes*. New York: Marlowe and Company, 2007.

Colberg, Sheri R. *The 7 Step Diabetes Fitness Plan: Living Well and Being Fit with Diabetes, No Matter Your Weight*. New York: Marlowe and Company, 2006.

Daniels, Dianne M. *Exercises for Osteoporosis: A Safe and Effective Way to Build Bone Density and Muscle Strength*. Revised ed. Long Island City, NY: Hatherleigh Press, 2005.

Dychtwald, Ken. *Age Power: How the 21st Century Will Be Ruled by the New Old*. New York: Tarcher, 2001.

Evans, William J., and Gerald Couzens. *AstroFit: The Astronaut Program for Anti-Aging*. New York: Free Press, 2003.

Joseph, James, Daniel Nadeau, and Anne Underwood. *The Color Code: A Revolutionary Eating Plan for Optimum Health*. New York: Hyperion, 2003.

Kimble, Melvin A., ed., et al. *Aging, Spirituality, and Religion: A Handbook*. Minneapolis: Augsburg Fortress, 2004.

Koenig, Harold, and Harvey Cohen. *The Link Between Religion and Health: Psychoneuroimmunology and the Faith Factor*. New York: Oxford University Press, 2002.

Lindauer, Martin S. *Aging, Creativity, and Art: A Positive Perspective on Late-Life Development.* New York: Klewer Academic/Plenum Publishers, 2003.

Lipschitz, David A. *Breaking the Rules of Aging.* New ed. Washington, D.C.: Lifeline Press, 2005.

MacKenzie, Elizabeth R., ed. *Complementary and Alternative Medicine for Older Adults: Holistic Approaches to Healthy Aging.* New York: Springer, 2006.

Radin, Lisa, ed. *What If It's Not Alzheimer's: A Caregiver's Guide to Dementia.* Amherst, NY: Prometheus Books, 2003.

Roizen, Michael F., and Mehmet Oz. *YOU: The Owner's Manual: An Insider's Guide to the Body That Will Make You Healthier and Younger.* New York: HarperCollins, 2005.

Snowdon, David. *Aging with Grace: What the Nun Study Teaches Us About Leading Longer, Healthier, and More Meaningful Lives.* Reprint ed. New York: Bantam, 2002.

Stein, Richard. *Outliving Heart Disease: The 10 New Rules for Prevention and Treatment.* New York: Newmarket Press, 2006.

Selected References

Introduction

Beare, S. (2006). *50 secrets of the world's longest living people*. New York: Marlowe and Company, 2006, 1–45.

Gruenewald, T. L., Seeman, T. E., Ryff, C. D., Karlamangla, A. S., and Singer, B. H. (2006). Combinations of biomarkers predictive of later life mortality. *Proc Natl Acad Sci USA*, 103(38), 14158–63.

Karasik, D., Demissie, S., Cupples, L. A., and Kiel, D. P. (2005). Disentangling the genetic determinants of human aging: Biological age as an alternative to the use of survival measures. *J Gerontol*, 60A(5), 574–87.

Kim, M. J., and Morley, J. E. (2005). The hormonal fountains of youth: Myth or reality? *J Endocrinol Invest*, 28(Suppl. 11), 5–14.

Step 1

Avogaro, A., Watanabe, R. M., Dall'Arche, A., et al. (2004). Acute alcohol consumption improves insulin action without affecting insulin secretion in type 2 diabetic subjects. *Diab Care*, 27(6), 1369–74.

Bottiglieri, T. (1996). Folate, vitamin B_{12}, and neuropsychiatric disorders. *Nutrition Rev*, 54(12), 382–90.

Cordova, A. C., Jackson, L. S., Berke-Schlessel, D. W., and Sumpio, B. E. (2005). The cardiovascular protective effect of red wine. *J Am Coll Surg*, 200(3), 428–39.

Couzin, J. (2006). Women's health: Study yields murky signals on low-fat diets and disease. *Science*, 311(5762), 755.

Dufresne, C. J., and Farnworth, E. R. (2001). A review of latest research findings on the health promotion properties of tea. *J Nutri Biochem*, 12(7), 404–21.

Farr, S. A., Poon, H. F., Dogrukol-Ak, D., et al. (2003). The antioxidants alpha-lipoic acid and N-acetylcysteine reverse memory impairment and brain oxidative stress in aged SAMP8 mice. *J Neurochem*, 84(5), 1173–83.

Fisher, A., and Morley, J. E. (2002). Antiaging medicine: The good, the bad, and the ugly. *J Gerontol*, 57(10), M636–M639.

Fisher, N. D, Sorond, F. A., and Hollenberg, N. K. (2006). Cocoa flavanols and brain perfusion. *J Cardiovasc Pharmacol*, 47(Suppl. 2), S210–S214.

Freund-Levi, Y., Eriksdotter-Honhagen, M., Cederholm, T., et al. (2006). Omega-3 fatty acid treatment in 174 patients with mild to moderate Alzheimer disease: OmegAD study. *Arch Neurol*, 63(10), 1402–8.

Gammack, J. K., and Morley, J. E. (2004). Anti-aging medicine—the good, the bad, and the ugly. *Clin Geriatr Med*, 20(2), 157–77.

Gotshalk, L. A., Volek, J. S., and Staron, R. S., et al. (2002). Creatine supplementation improves muscular performance in older men. *Med Sci Sports Exerc*, 34(3), 537–43.

Hathcock, J. N., Shao, A., Vieth, R., and Heaney, R. (2007). Risk assessment for vitamin D. *Am J Clin Nutr*, 85(1), 6–18.

Kris-Etherton, P. M., Harris, W. S., and Appel, L. J. American Heart Association. Nutrition Committee. (2002). Fish consumption, fish oil, omega-3 fatty acids, and cardiovascular disease. *Circ*, 106(21), 2747–57.

Launer, L. J., and Kalmijn, S. (1988). Anti-oxidants and cognitive function: A review of clinical and epidemiologic studies. *J Neural Transm*, 53, 1–8.

Lindeman, R. D., Romero, L. J., Liang, H. C., et al. (2002). Do elderly persons need to be encouraged to drink more fluids? *J Gerontol*, 55(7), M361–M365.

Lopez-Garcia, E., Schulze, M. B., Meigs, J. B., et al. (2005). Consumption of trans fatty acids is related to plasma biomarkers of inflammation and endothelial dysfunction. *J Nutr*, 135(3), 562–66.

Mozaffarian, D., and Rimm, E. B. (2006). Fish intake, contaminants, and human health: Evaluating the risks and the benefits. *JAMA*, 296(15), 1885–99.

Ott, B. R., and Owens, N. J. (1998). Complementary and alternative medicines for Alzheimer's disease. *J Geriatr Psych Neuro*, 11(4), 163–73.

Rimm, E. B., Klatsky, A., Grobbee, D., et al. (1996). Review of moderate alcohol consumption and reduced risk of coronary heart disease: Is the effect due to beer, wine, or spirits? *Brit Med J*, 312(7033), 731–36.

Thun, M. J., Peto, R., Lopez, A. D., et al. (1997). Alcohol consumption and mortality among middle-aged and elderly U.S. adults. *New Engl J Med*, 337(24), 1705–14.

Wilson, M. M, and Morley, J. E. (2003). Aging and energy balance. *J Appl Physiol*, 95(4), 1728–36.

Zairis, M. N., Ambrose J. A., Lyras A. G., et al. (2004). C-reactive protein, moderate alcohol consumption, and long-term prognosis after successful coronary stenting: Four-year results from the GENERATION study. *Heart*, 90(4), 419–24.

Zern, T. L., and Fernandez, M. L. (2005). Cardioprotective effects of dietary polyphenols. *J Nutr*, 135(10), 2291–94.

Step 2

Berk, D. R., Hubert, H. B., and Fries, J. F. (2006). Associations of changes in exercise level with subsequent disability among seniors: A 16-year longitudinal study. *J Gerontol*, 61(1), 97–102.

Christmas, C., and Andersen, R. A. (2000). Exercise and older patients: Guidelines for the clinician. *J Am Geriatr Soc*, 48(7), 318–24.

Colberg, S. R. (2006). The impact of exercise on insulin action in type 2 diabetes mellitus: Relationship to prevention and control. *Insulin*, 1(3), 85–98.

Dunn, A. L., Trivedi, M. H., Kampert, J. B., et al. (2005). Exercise treatment for depression: Efficacy and dose response. *Am J Prev Med*, 28(1), 1–8.

Evans, W. J. (1999). Exercise training guidelines for the elderly. *Med Sci Sports Exerc*, 31(1), 12–17.

Fletcher, G. F., Balady, G. J., Amsterdam, E. A., et al. (2001). Exercise standards for testing and training: A statement for healthcare professionals from the American Heart Association, *Circ*, 104(14), 1694–1740.

Haapanen, N., Miilunpalo, S., Vuori, I., et al. (1996). Characteristics of leisure time physical activity associated with decreased risk of premature all-cause and cardiovascular disease mortality in middle-aged men. *Am J Epidemiol*, 143(9), 870–80.

Hood, S., and Northcote, R. J. (1999). Cardiac assessment of veteran endurance athletes: A 12-year follow-up study. *Br J Sports Med*, 33(4), 239–43.

Hubert, H. B., and Fries, J. F. (1994). Predictors of physical disability after 50: Six-year longitudinal study in a runners club and a university population. *Ann Epidemiol*, 4(4), 285–94.

Larson, E. B., Wang, L., Bowen, J. D., et al. (2006). Exercise is associated with reduced risk for incident dementia among persons 65 years of age and older. *Ann Intern Med*, 144(2), 73–81.

Mazzeo, R. S., Cavanagh, P., Evans, W. J., et al. (1998). ACSM position stand on exercise and physical activity for older adults. *Med Sci Sports Exerc*, 30(6), 992–1008.

Morley, J. E., and Reese, S. S. (1989). Clinical implications of the aging heart. *Am J Med*, 86(1), 77–86.

Patel, K. V., Coppin, A. K., Manini, T. M., et al. (2006). Midlife physical activity and mobility in older age: The InCHIANTI study. *Am J Prev Med*, 31(3), 217–24.

Pollock, M. L., Franklin, B. A., Balady, G. J., et al. (2002). AHA Science Advisory. Resistance exercise in individuals with and without cardio-vascular disease: Benefits, rationale, safety, and prescription: An advisory from the Committee on Exercise, Rehabilitation, and Prevention, Council on Clinical Cardiology, American Heart Association. *Circ*, 101(7), 828–33.

Shephard, R. J. (2000). Does insistence on medical clearance inhibit adoption of physical activity in the elderly? *J Aging Phys Activity*, 8(4), 301–11.

Step 3

Farr, S. A., Banks, W. A., Uezu, K., et al. (2004). DHEAS improves learning and memory in aged SAMP8 mice but not in diabetic mice. *Life Sci*, 75(23), 2775–85.

Horani, M. H, and Morley, J. E. (2004). Hormonal fountains of youth. *Clin Geriatr Med*, 20(2), 275–92.

Morley, J. E. (2003). Hormones and the aging process. *J Am Geriatr Soc*, 51(Suppl. 7), S333–S337.

Morley, J. E. (2001). Testosterone replacement in older men and women. *J Gend Specif Med*, 4(2), 49–53.

Morley, J. E., Haren, M. T., Kim, M. J., et al. (2005). Testosterone, aging and quality of life. *J Endocrinol Invest*, 28(Suppl. 3), 76–80.

Morley, J. E., and Perry III, H. M. (2003). Andropause: An old concept in new clothing. *Clin Geriatr Med*, 19(3), 507–28.

Rossouw, J. E., Anderson, G. L., Prentice, R. L., et al. (2002). Risks and benefits of estrogen plus progestin in healthy postmenopausal women: Principal results from the Women's Health Initiative randomized controlled trial. *JAMA*, 288(3), 321–33.

Travison, T. G., Morley, J. E., Araujo, A. B., et al. (2006). The relationship between libido and testosterone levels in aging men. *J Clin Endocrinol Metab*, 91(7), 2509–13.

Step 4

Banks, W. A., and Morley, J. E. (2003). Memories are made of this: Recent advances in understanding cognitive impairments and dementia. *J Gerontol*, 58(4), 314–21.

Banks, W. A., Pagliari, P., Nakaoke, R., and Morley, J. E. (2005). Effects of a behaviorally active antibody on the brain uptake and clearance of amyloid beta proteins. *Peptides*, 26(2), 287–94.

Blazer, D. G. (2003). Depression in late life: Review and commentary. *J Gerontol*, 58(3), 249–65.

Broe, G. A., et al. (1998). Health habits and risk of cognitive impairment and dementia in old age: A prospective study on the effects of exercise, smoking, and alcohol consumption. *Austral New Zeal J Pub Health*, 22(5), 621–23.

Farr, S. A., Poon, H. F., Dogrukol-Ak D., et al. (2003). The antioxidants alpha-lipoic acid and N-acetylcysteine reverse memory impairment and brain oxidative stress in aged SAMP8 mice. *J Neurochem*, 84(5), 1173–83.

Fisher, N. D., Sorond, F. A., and Hollenberg, N. K. (2006). Cocoa flavanols and brain perfusion. *J Cardiovasc Pharmacol*, 47(Suppl. 2), S210–14.

Freund-Levi, Y., Eriksdotter-Honhagen, M., Cederholm, T., et al. (2006). Omega-3 fatty acid treatment in 174 patients with mild to moderate Alzheimer disease: OmegAD study. *Arch Neurol*, 63(10), 1402–8.

Grossberg, G. T., and Desai, A. K. (2003). Management of Alzheimer's disease. *J Gerontol*, 58(4), 331–53.

Johsi, S., and Morley, J. E. (2006). Cognitive impairment. *Med Clin North Am*, 90(5), 769–87.

Kado, D. M., Karlamangla, A. S., Huang, M. H., et al. (2005). Homocysteine versus the vitamins folate, B6, and B12 as predictors of cognitive function and decline in older high-functioning adults: MacArthur Studies of Successful Aging. *Am J Med*, 118(2), 161–67.

Koster A., Bosma H., Kempen G. I., et al. (2006). Socioeconomic differences in incident depression in older adults: The role of psychosocial factors, physical health status, and behavioral factors. *J Psychosom Res*, 61(5), 619–27.

Kramer, A. F. (2006). Exercise, cognition, and the aging brain. *J Appl Physiol*, 101(4), 1237–42.

Larson, E. B., Wang, L., Bowen, J. D., et al. (2006). Exercise is associated with reduced risk for incident dementia among persons 65 years of age and older. *Ann Intern Med*, 144(2), 73–81.

Morris, M. C., Evans, D. A., Tangney C. C., et al. (2006). Associations of vegetable and fruit consumption with age-related cognitive change. *Neurology*, 67(8), 1370–76.

Oken, B. S., Storzbach, D. M., and Kaye, J. A. (1998). The efficacy of Ginkgo biloba on cognitive function in Alzheimer's disease. *Arch Neurol*, 55(11), 1409–15.

Small, G. (2004). *The memory prescription*. New York: Hyperion.

van Crevel, H., van Gool, W. A., and Walstra, G. J. M. (1999). Early diagnosis of dementia: Which tests are indicated? What are their costs? *J Neurol*, 246(2), 73–78.

Step 5

Dirks, A. J., and Leeuwenburgh, C. (2006). Tumor necrosis factor alpha signaling in skeletal muscle: Effects of age and caloric restriction. *J Nutr Biochem*, 17(8), 501–8.

Goodpaster, B. H., Park, S. W., Harris, T. B., et al. (2006). The loss of skeletal muscle strength, mass, and quality in older adults: The health, aging and body composition study. *J Gerontol*, 61(10), 1059–64.

Holmes, S. (2006). Barriers to effective nutritional care for older adults. *Nurs Stand*, 21(3), 50–54.

Jagust, W., Harvey, D., Mungas, D., and Haan, M. (2005). Central obesity and the aging brain. *Arch Neurol*, 62(10), 1545–48.

Morley, J. E. (2001). Anorexia, sarcopenia, and aging. *Nutrition*, 17(7–8), 660–63.

Morley, J. E. (2001). Anorexia, body composition, and aging. *Curr Opin Clin Nutr Metab Care*, 4(1), 9–13.

Morley, J. E., and Baumgartner, R. N. (2004) Cytokine-related aging process. *J Gerontol*, 59(9), M924–M929.

Morley J. E., Thomas D. R., and Wilson M. M. (2006). Cachexia: Pathophysiology and clinical relevance. *Am J Clin Nutr*, 83(4), 735–43.

Paddon-Jones, D. (2006). Interplay of stress and physical inactivity on muscle loss: Nutritional countermeasures. *J Nutr*, 136(8), 2123–26.

Schneider, S. M., Al-Jaouni, R., Pivot, X., et al. (2002). Lack of adaptation to severe malnutrition in elderly patients. *Clin Nutr*, 21(6), 499–504.

Turner, K. W. (2006). Weight status and participation in senior center activities. *Fam Community Health*, 29(4), 279–87.

Step 6

American Diabetes Association. (1998). Consensus development conference on the diagnosis of coronary heart disease in people with diabetes. *Diab Care*, 21(9), 1551–59.

Banning, M. (2005). The role of omega-3-fatty acids in the prevention of cardiac events. *Br J Nurs*, 14(9), 503–8.

Danaei, G., Lawes, C. M., Vander Hoorn, S., et al. (2006). Global and regional mortality from ischaemic heart disease and stroke attributable to higher-than-optimum blood glucose concentration: Comparative risk assessment. *Lancet*, 368(9548), 1651–59.

Diabetes Prevention Program Research Group, Crandall, J., Schade, D., et al. (2006). The influence of age on the effects of lifestyle modification and metformin in prevention of diabetes. *J Gerontol*, 61(10), 1075–81.

Donnelly, R. (2005). Managing cardiovascular risk in patients with diabetes. *Br J Diabetes Vasc Dis*, 5(6), 325–29.

Heiss, C., Schroeter, H., Balzer, J., et al. (2006). Endothelial function, nitric oxide, and cocoa flavanols. *J Cardiovasc Pharmacol*, 47(Suppl. 2), S128–S135.

Jacobson, T. A. (2006). Secondary prevention of coronary artery disease with omega-3 fatty acids. *Am J Cardiol*, 98(4A), 61i–70i.

Knowler, W. C., Barrett-Connor E., Fowler, S. E., et al. (2002). Reduction in the incidence of type 2 diabetes with lifestyle intervention or metformin. *N Engl J Med*, 346(6), 393–403.

Kris-Etherton, P. M., Harris, W. S., and Appel, L. J. American Heart Association. Nutrition Committee. (2002). Fish consumption, fish oil, omega-3 fatty acids, and cardiovascular disease. *Circ*, 106(21), 2747–57.

Michael, K. M., and Shaughnessy, M. (2006). Stroke prevention and management in older adults. *J Cardiovasc Nurs*, 21(5 Suppl 1), S21–S26.

Morley, J. E., and Reese, S. S. (1989). Clinical implications of the aging heart. *Am J Med*, 86(1), 77–86.

Mukamal, K. J., Chiuve, S. E., and Rimm, E. B. (2006). Alcohol consumption and risk for coronary heart disease in men with healthy lifestyles. *Arch Intern Med*, 166(19), 2145–50.

Oh, R. C., Beresford, S. A., and Lafferty, W. E. (2006). The fish in secondary prevention of heart disease (FISH) survey—primary care physicians and omega-3 fatty acid prescribing behaviors. J *Am Board Fam Med*, 19(5), 459–67.

Orchard, T. J., Temprosa, M., Goldberg, R., et al. (2005). The effect of metformin and intensive lifestyle intervention on the metabolic syndrome: The Diabetes Prevention Program randomized trial. *Ann Intern Med*, 142(8), 611–19.

Rich, M. W. (2006). Heart failure in older adults. *Med Clin North Am*, 90(5), 863–85.

Safar, M. E., Smulyan, H. (2006). Blood pressure components in clinical hypertension. *J Clin Hypertens*, 8(9), 659–66.

Vakkilainen, J., Steiner, G., Ansquer, J. C., et al. (2003). Relationships between low-density lipoprotein particle size, plasma lipoproteins, and progression of coronary artery disease: The Diabetes Atherosclerosis Intervention Study (DAIS). *Circ*, 107(13), 1733–37.

Vinson, J. A., Proch, J., Bose, P., et al. (2006). Chocolate is a powerful ex vivo and in vivo antioxidant, an antiatherosclerotic agent in an animal model, and a significant contributor to antioxidants in the European and American diets. *J Agric Food Chem*, 54(21), 8071–76.

Step 7

Argiles, J. M., Busquets, S., Felipe, A., and Lopez-Soriano, F. J. (2006). Muscle wasting in cancer and ageing: Cachexia versus sarcopenia. *Adv Gerontol*, 18, 39–54.

Cohen, H. J. (2006). Cancer survivorship and ageing—a double whammy. *Lancet Oncol*, 7(11), 882–83.

Costa, G. J., Fernandes, A. L., Pereira, J. R., Curtis, J. R., and Santoro, I. L. (2006). Survival rates and tolerability of platinum-based chemotherapy regimens for elderly patients with non-small-cell lung cancer (NSCLC). *Lung Cancer*, 53(2), 171–76.

Greco, K. (2006). Cancer screening in older adults in an era of genomics and longevity. *Semin Oncol Nurs*, 22(1), 10–19.

Guarneri, V., and Conte, P. F. (2004). The curability of breast cancer and the treatment of advanced disease. *Eur J Nucl Med Mol Imaging*, 31(Suppl. 1), S149–S161.

Kamangar, F., Dores, G. M., and Anderson, W. F. (2006). Patterns of cancer incidence, mortality, and prevalence across five continents: Defining priorities to reduce cancer disparities in different geographic regions of the world. *J Clin Oncol*, 24(14), 2137–50.

Keller, K. L., Fenske, N. A., and Glass, L. F. (1997). Cancer of the skin in the older patient. *Clin Geriatr Med*, 13(2), 339–61.

Kleinman, K. P., and McKinlay, J. B. (2000). Prostate cancer: How much do we know and how do we know it? *Aging Male*, 3(3), 115–23.

Kuriki, K., and Tajima, K. (2006). The increasing incidence of colorectal cancer and the preventive strategy in Japan. *Asian Pac J Cancer Prev*, 7(3), 495–501.

Smith, R. A., Cokkinides, V., and Eyre, H. J. (2006). American Cancer Society guidelines for the early detection of cancer, 2006. *CA Cancer J Clin*, 56(1), 11–25.

White, H. K., and Cohen, H. J. (2006). The older cancer patient. *Med Clin North Am*, 90(5), 967–82.

Witherby, S. M., and Muss, H. B. (2006). Managing early-stage breast cancer in your older patients. *Oncology*, 20(9), 1003–12.

Wolpowitz, D., and Gilchrest, B. A. (2006). The vitamin D questions: How much do you need and how should you get it? *J Am Acad Dermatol*, 54(2), 301–17.

Step 8

Distler, J., and Anguelouch, A. (2006). Evidence-based practice: Review of clinical evidence on the efficacy of glucosamine and chondroitin in the treatment of osteoarthritis. *J Am Acad Nurse Pract*, 18(10), 487–93.

Feskanich, D., Willett, W. C., and Colditz, G. A. (2003). Calcium, vitamin D, milk consumption, and hip fractures: A prospective study among postmenopausal women. *Am J Clin Nutr*, 77(2), 504–11.

Frassetto, L. A., Todd, K. M., Morris, R. C., Jr., et al. (2000). Worldwide incidence of hip fracture in elderly women: Relation to consumption of animal and vegetable foods. *J Gerontol*, 55(10), M585-M592.

Grimes, D. S. (2006). Are statins analogues of vitamin D? *Lancet*, 368(9529), 83–86.

Kerstetter, J. E., O'Brien, K. O., Caseria, D. M., et al. (2005). The impact of dietary protein on calcium absorption and kinetic measures of bone turnover in women. *J Clin Endocrinol Metab*, 90(1), 26–31.

Kerstetter, J. E., O'Brien, K. O., and Insogna, K. L. (2003). Low protein intake: The impact on calcium and bone homeostasis in humans. *J Nutr*, 133(3), 855S–861S.

Martin, K., Fontaine, K. R., Nicklas, B. J., et al. (2001). Weight loss and exercise walking reduce pain and improve physical functioning in overweight postmenopausal women with knee osteoarthritis. *J Clin Rheumatol*, 7(4), 219–23.

Mikesky, A. E., Mazzuca, S. A., Brandt, K. D., et al. (2006). Effects of strength training on the incidence and progression of knee osteoarthritis. *Arthritis Rheum*, 55(5), 690–99, 2006.

Munger, R. G., Cerhan, J. R., and Chiu, B. C. (1999). Prospective study of dietary protein intake and risk of hip fracture in postmenopausal women. *Am J Clin Nutr*, 69(1), 147–52.

Perry III, H. M., and Morley, J. E. (2001). Osteoporosis in men: Are we ready to diagnose and treat? *Curr Rheumatol Rep*, 3(3), 240–44.

Promislow, J. H., Goodman-Gruen, D., Slymen, D. J., et al. (2002). Protein consumption and bone mineral density in the elderly: The Rancho Bernardo Study. *Am J Epidemiol*, 155(7), 636–44.

Ryder, K. M., Shorr, R. I., Tylavsky, F. A., et al. (2006). Correlates of use of antifracture therapy in older women with low bone mineral density. *J Gen Intern Med*, 21(6), 636–41.

Sellmeyer, D. E., Stone, K. L., Sebastian, A., et al. (2001). A high ratio of dietary animal to vegetable protein increases the rate of bone loss and the risk of fracture in postmenopausal women. *Am J Clin Nutr*, 73(1), 118–22.

Vignon, E., Valat, J. P., Rossignol, M., et al. (2006). Osteoarthritis of the knee and hip and activity: A systematic international review and synthesis (OASIS). *Joint Bone Spine*, 73(4), 442–55.

Step 9

Argiles, J. M., Busquets, S., Felipe, A., and Lopez-Soriano, F. J. (2006). Muscle wasting in cancer and ageing: Cachexia versus sarcopenia. *Adv Gerontol*, 18, 39–54.

Bartali, B., Frongillo, E. A, Bandinelli, S., et al. (2006). Low nutrient intake is an essential component of frailty in older persons. *J Gerontol*, 61(6), 589–93.

Baumgartner, R. N., Wayne, S. J., Waters, D. L., et al. (2004). Sarcopenic obesity predicts instrumental activities of daily living disability in the elderly. *Obes Res*, 12(12), 1995–2004.

Bischoff, H. A., Staehelin, H. B., Willett, W. C. (2006). The effect of undernutrition in the development of frailty in older persons. *J Gerontol*, 61(6), 585–89.

Blaum, C. S., Xue, Q. L., Michelon, E., et al. (2005). The association between obesity and the frailty syndrome in older women: The Women's Health and Aging Studies. *J Am Geriatr Soc*, 53(6), 927–34.

Freedman, V. A., Hodgson, N., Lynn, J., et al. (2006). Promoting declines in the prevalence of late-life disability: comparisons of three potentially high-impact interventions. *Milbank Q*, 84(3), 493–520.

Kotz, C. M., Wang, C., Teske, J. A, et al. (2006). Orexin A mediation of time spent moving in rats: Neural mechanism. *Neuroscience*, 142(1), 29–36.

Levine, J. A., Eberhardt, N. L., and Jensen, M. D. (1999). Role of nonexercise activity thermogenesis in resistance to fat gain in humans. *Science*, 283(5399), 212–14.

Manini, T. M., Everhart, J. E., Patel, K. V., et al. (2006). Daily activity energy expenditure and mortality among older adults. *JAMA*, 296(2), 171–79.

Morley, J. E. (2002). A fall is a major event in the life of an older person. *J Gerontol*, 57(8), M492–M495.

Morley, J. E., Perry III, H. M., and Miller, D. K. (2002). Something about frailty. *J Gerontol*, 57(11), M698–M670.

Morley, J. E. (2004). The top 10 hot topics in aging. *J Gerontol*, 59(1), 24–33.

Morley, J. E., Kim, M. J., Haren, M. T., et al. (2005). Frailty and the aging male. *Aging Male*, 8(3–4), 135–40.

Morley, J. E., Thomas, D. R., and Wilson, M. M. (2006). Cachexia: Pathophysiology and clinical relevance. *Am J Clin Nutr*, 83(4), 735–43.

Paganelli, R., Di Iorio, A., Cherubini, A., et al. (2006). Frailty of older age: The role of the endocrine—immune interaction. *Curr Pharm Des*, 12(24), 3147–59.

Step 10

Fick, D. M., Cooper, J. W., Wade, W. E., Waller, J. L., Maclean, J. R., and Beers, M. H. (2003). Updating the Beers criteria for potentially inappropriate medication use in older adults: Results of a US consensus panel of experts. *Arch Intern Med*, 163(22), 2716–24.

Fretheim, A. (2003). Back to thiazide-diuretics for hypertension: Reflections after a decade of irrational prescribing. *BMC Fam Pract*, 4, 19.

Onder, G., Landi, F., Liperoti, R., et al. (2005). Impact of inappropriate drug use among hospitalized older adults. *Eur J Clin Pharmacol*, 61(5–6), 453–59.

Sheikh, J. I., Yesavage, J. A, Brooks II, J. O., et al. (1991). Proposed factor structure of the Geriatric Depression Scale. *Int Psychogeriatr*, 3(1), 23–28.

Starfield, B. (2000). Is U.S. health really the best in the world? *JAMA*, 284(4), 483–85.

Tariq, S. H., Tumosa, N., Chibnall, J. T., Perry III, H. M., and Morley, J. E. (2006). Comparison of the Saint Louis University mental status examination and the mini-mental state examination for detecting dementia and mild neurocognitive disorder—a pilot study. *Am J Geriatr Psych*, 14(11), 900–910.

Walter, L. C., and Covinsky, K. E. (2001). Cancer screening in elderly patients: a framework for individualized decision making. *JAMA*, 285(21), 2750–56, 2001.

Xie, F., Petitti, D. B., and Chen, W. (2005). Prescribing patterns for antihypertensive drugs after the Antihypertensive and Lipid-Lowering Treatment to Prevent Heart Attack Trial: Report of experience in a health maintenance organization. *Am J Hypertens*, 18(4 Pt. 1), 464–69.

Conclusion

Lo, B., Quill T., and Tulsky, J., for the ACP-ASIM End-of-Life Care Consensus Panel. (1999). Discussing palliative care with patients. *Ann Intern Med*, 130(9), 744–49.

Lo, B., Ruston, D., Kates, L. W., et al. (2002). Discussing religious and spiritual issues at the end of life. A practical guide for physicians. *JAMA*, 287(6), 749–54.

Poon, H. F., Joshi, G., Sultana, R., et al. (2004). Antisense directed at the Abeta region of APP decreases brain oxidative markers in aged senescence accelerated mice. *Brain Res,* 1018(1), 86–96.

Shanahan, M. J., and Hofer, S. M. (2005). Social context in gene-environment interactions: Retrospect and prospect. *J Gerontol*, 60(Spec No 1), 65–76.

Steinhauser, K. E., Christakis, N. A., Clipp, E. C., et al. (2000). Factors considered important at the end of life by patients, family, physicians, and other care providers. *JAMA*, 284(19), 2476–2482.

Zahn, J. M., Sonu, R., Vogel, H., et al. (2006). Transcriptional profiling of aging in human muscle reveals a common aging signature. *PLoS Genet*, 2(7), e115.

Index

About the Authors

John E. Morley, M.B., B.Ch., known internationally as a gerontological researcher, clinician, and educator, is the director of Saint Louis University's (SLU) Division of Geriatric Medicine and the Dammert Professor of Gerontology, as well as the director of the Geriatric Research, Education, and Clinical Center at the Saint Louis Veterans Administration Medical Center. SLU's Division of Geriatric Medicine, which he founded in 1989, is ranked as one of the top ten geriatric programs in the country, and he is routinely included in the Best Doctors of America. In addition to consulting for major pharmaceutical companies, such as Amgen, GTx, PAR Pharmaceuticals, and Merck, he is the chief scientific officer for Edunn Biotechnology Company, which is doing human studies on the Alzheimer's drug he developed. With Mattern Pharmaceuticals he has also developed a nasal testosterone for both men and women.

A true expert in his field, he has published twenty-one professional medical books for which he has been an editor and a contributor, including *Geriatric Nutrition, Science of Geriatrics, Medical Care in the Nursing Home,* and *Principles and Practice of Geriatric Medicine.* He has also published more than a thousand papers, and his scientific work has been cited over 20,000 times. He has also been an editor for all of the Merck Manuals, including their popular home editions, as well as for the *Journal of the American Medical Directors Association* and previously the *Journals of Gerontology: Medical Sciences.* A founder and major contributor to *Aging Successfully,* a collaborative newsletter of Saint Louis University and others, he has received innumerable awards for his work, including ones from the American Geriatrics Society, Gerontology Society of America, American Society for Clinical Nutrition, American Dietetic Association, Veterans Administration, and the Ipsen Longevity Award. He is happily married and has five grandchildren, who keep him busy.

Sheri R. Colberg, Ph.D., is an exercise physiologist and professor of exercise science at Old Dominion University in Norfolk, Virginia. Since attaining her undergraduate degree from Stanford University and her doctorate from the University of California, Berkeley, she has authored well over one hundred research and educational articles and several book chapters on exercise, diabetes, and physical activity, as well as four books for professional and lay audiences: *The Diabetic Athlete*, *Diabetes-Free Kids*, *The 7 Step Diabetes Fitness Plan*, and *50 Secrets of the Longest Living People with Diabetes*. A funded diabetes researcher, she is a Fellow of the American College of Sports Medicine and a professional member of the American Diabetes Association. In addition to professional training, she has almost four decades of practical experience as a type 1 diabetic exerciser, as well as living and aging well with a chronic health condition. She currently resides in Virginia Beach, Virginia, with her husband and their three boys. An avid recreational exerciser, she enjoys swimming, biking, running, walking, tennis, weight training, soccer, hiking, yard work, and a variety of other fitness activities.